Health and Social Care in the Digital World

T0144126

Health and Social Care in the Digital World

Meeting the Challenge for Primary Care

Nigel Starey

Retired Family Doctor and Academic GP
and
Advisor
Care Quality Commission
United Kingdom

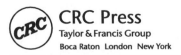

CRC Press
Taylor & Francis Group
Boca Raton London New York

CRC Press is an imprint of the
Taylor & Francis Group, an **informa** business

First edition published 2020
by CRC Press
6000 Broken Sound Parkway NW, Suite 300, Boca Raton, FL 33487-2742

and by CRC Press
2 Park Square, Milton Park, Abingdon, Oxon, OX14 4RN

© 2020 Taylor & Francis Group, LLC

CRC Press is an imprint of Taylor & Francis Group, LLC

Library of Congress Cataloging-in-Publication Data

Names: Starey, Nigel, author.
Title: Health and social care in the digital world : meeting the challenge for primary care / Nigel Starey.
Description: First edition. | Boca Raton : CRC Press, 2020. | Includes bibliographical references and index. | Summary: "This provocative and timely book examines the current state of primary care practice and outlines a new vision for the delivery of primary care services, primarily in the UK but also internationally. Encouraging a social compact between citizens, governments and the providers of care, the book describes how this will necessitate a redesign of the welfare sector to ensure it is 'fit for purpose' in the digital world. It explores the respective roles of the inverse care law and the rule of halves, systems theory and learning organisations, mutuality and active citizenship, and how these can be applied to improve service delivery. Key features: Offers an alternative approach to thinking and a challenge to leaders within primary care and to those with administrative responsibility for the sector. Reflects the multiple challenges facing primary care, including the rise in frail elderly patients, increasing multi-morbidities, the impact of changing demography with migration and much more. Sets these challenges in a context of increasing workforce pressures, including changing attitudes to professionalism, burnout and recruitment difficulties Outlines a road map for improvement responding to current challenges around social care as well as digital/e-health. Aimed at, and written for, all those committed to improving the future of the primary care sector in the UK and internationally, this important book will be of interest to students, clinicians, managers, commissioners, policy makers and service users"-- Provided by publisher.
Identifiers: LCCN 2019057834 | ISBN 9780367858261 (paperback) | ISBN 9780367858391 (hardback) | ISBN 9781003031079 (ebook)
Subjects: MESH: Great Britain. National Health Service. | Primary Health Care--organization & administration | Social Welfare | Health Care Reform | United Kingdom
Classification: LCC RA418.5.P6 | NLM W 84.6 FA1 | DDC 362.1/0425--dc23
LC record available at https://lccn.loc.gov/2019057834

ISBN: 978-0-367-85839-1 (hbk)
ISBN: 978-0-367-85826-1 (pbk)
ISBN: 978-1-003-03107-9 (ebk)

Typeset in Minion
by Nova Techset Private Limited, Bengaluru & Chennai, India

Contents

Foreword

It has been twenty-five years since primary care last received such attention. Those with long memories can recall a document by the Department of Health pushing towards a primary care–led National Health Service (NHS) in the 1990s. Now the coming of primary care networks has brought us primary care's very own Five-Year plan with 20,000 more staff and new kinds of services across the community.

In this time of new anxiety about the future, this book represents a valuable contribution on the scope for local initiatives. It deals with issues which only GPs and their teams can deal with. Primary care is not just a sum of activities; it must have its own priorities and a sense of its own identity. Public plans and reports cannot deal with the subjective elements of values – issues about "mutuality" and "trust".

The first key from author Nigel Starey is *active citizenship*. This is about a shared commitment between patient and professional to improve health. Lifestyle improvements need motivation and they have to be followed up over time. The new contract document calls it anticipatory care, which could be about identifying patients with high risk. This value points to the need for longer-term relationship-building with patients. Values point to activity that represents the GP's own choice about how to use time.

The second key is *redefined professionalism*. Starey coins the useful term "pseudo team", which is there on paper but has little mutual learning or contact. Real teamwork is about shared objectives and regular review of achievements against objectives. The wider team has a shared responsibility for safeguarding and for care programmes.

The third key is *mutuality*. The out-of-hospital sector can operate as a learning system: "a system which is continually expanding its capacity to create its own future, not merely to survive through adapting to circumstance".

Finally, there is *organisational integration*. This involves a shared information base and a shared commitment to personal care. For the future there has to be greater integration within the practice and integration with staff across the network.

Near the start of the book, Starey sets out the key problems that lead to primary care being a "burning platform": overwork, increased patient load and staffing deficiencies. But he is unusually realistic in his view that more funding and more staffing are not necessarily the answers. General practice at present is a "1940s model which is no longer fit for our twenty-first century 'digital' age". Unless we move towards a new model, funding is simply going to grant a short rest from the current malfunctions before they return with more activity and more management problems. The NHS may soon look "like a cuckoo in the nest consuming more and more of the nation's resources at the expense of other competing priorities".

The book comes after the Care Quality Commission's report on general practice [1]. This had much good news about general practice. By 2017, 90 percent of the population was attending practices that were either good or outstanding, and practices in need of improvement had shown positive change. The weakest results were in London. Out of 1254 practices inspected, only 14 were outstanding and 17 percent of practices were inadequate or required improvement. In the North East, only 1 percent required improvement and 98 percent were good or outstanding, compared to 83 percent in London. Yorkshire and the South West were not far behind the North East. Thus, general practice does not have the usual North–South divide and is well placed to show initiative for citizens in more deprived areas.

Further back, GPs developed strength through the Royal College of General Practitioners (RCGP) and through their use of the Family Doctor Charter [2]. They showed remarkable initiative in developing IT systems and the Quality and Outcomes Framework (QOF) contract would have been impossible without the hard work of GPs in the 1980s and 1990s. They responded to new incentives in raising immunisation rates and developing cytology. Most of the gains in life expectancy from 1980 to 2010 were the result of primary care programmes, especially in coronary heart disease (CHD) and stroke prevention. Of course, there are problems in the rising numbers of patients, but this is because of success not failure. Patients want to use the service and 80 percent are satisfied with what they receive. Above all there is a cadre of specially trained primary care doctors – some 30,000, one of the largest group of primary care doctors worldwide. They work with the finest group of practice nurses and support staff. It is time for GPs to put forth a message of success and to show how they can develop the service further.

Nigel Starey has used his forty years of experience well in this book. It has a concise account of the problems, but it is mainly about solutions – and solutions that involve local initiatives by GP-led teams. The timetable for new service specifications may slip, but when that starts to happen, anticipatory care and personalisation can only develop local initiatives and local leadership. In essence, the call is for longer-term care programmes and partnerships with high-risk patients. For example, in COPD there are three key predictors of whether patients are likely to have serious exacerbations: a previous history, continuing to smoke and a missing sense of control over their disease [3]. Most emergency admissions with COPD are by patients with these problems. There are now simple measures of severity and disability in many disease areas.

The new personal communications network (PCN) space will give clinical directors the chance to develop a common vital digital base across practices – vital for care integration and for effective use of the time of the new staff. Clinical directors can also take the lead in developing outcome measures and research. Since pharmaceutical companies shifted most of their research on new drugs to hospitals, primary care has been starved of innovation. PCNs can do much to strengthen the evidence base for the expansion of primary care.

The new model as set out by Starey depends not just on plans from NHS England but also on initiatives by GPs and their teams. The book shows directions for initiatives and illustrates the key values which support it. It is a vital text for the new period of challenge.

Nick Bosanquet
Professor of Health Policy
Imperial College

REFERENCES

1. Care Quality Commission (CQC). 2017. The state of care in general practice 2014 to 2017.
2. Bosanquet N and Leese B. 1989. *Family Doctors and Economic Incentives*. Dartmouth Publishing, Aldershot.
3. Doward L, Scvedsater H, Whalley D et al. 2017. Salford Lung Study in chronic obstructive pulmonary disease (SLS COPD): Follow-up interviews on patient-centred care. *NPJ Primary Care Respiratory Medicine* 27(1):66.

Introduction: The burning platform

KEY MESSAGES

The book's key messages are presented right at the start, but the development and thinking which have led to them take up the rest of the book. They are presented here to make it absolutely clear where we are heading.

The current design of the British primary healthcare sector is no longer "fit for purpose" – we have a 1940s model which is no longer fit for our twenty-first century "digital" age. It has offered a national service with a uniform, "one size fits all" approach which lacks the flexibility of provision to make it fit for the digital age where the context within which the service is delivered is very different. The recommended redesign or transformation is based on four key elements and the following analysis makes the case for

1. Active citizenship
2. Redefined professionalism
3. Mutuality
4. Organisational integration

This means bringing together the elements of the existing National Health Service (NHS) "Mark 1", which have underpinned the success of the primary care sector for its first seventy years, together with the opportunities offered by the digital world we now live in.

These key messages and all that they imply form the material I consider in the rest of the book. I hope you will be energised by the analysis, engaged by the stories and examples, and inspired by the vision. While I recognise that we will all disagree about elements, or dimensions, of the design, I hope you find the book a positive force offering you and your family a glimpse of a more secure and healthier future.

"BURNING PLATFORMS"

These are very powerful drivers of strategic change [2]. They are what happens when

- There is a real and immediate crisis.
- There is a limited number of difficult and challenging choices or alternatives.
- Each of the choices is irreversible.
- Each choice has a high risk of failure.

The phrase comes from a real incident dating back to July 6, 1988. On that date the Piper Alpha oil rig in the North Sea exploded – the result of a failure to check some simple systems that had worked faultlessly for the previous decade. The explosion in turn caused a massive fire and 167 men died – the largest number killed in an offshore accident.

The scale of the blast was immense: the flames from the blaze shot 90 m in the air and apparently could be seen 100 km away. At first the workers locked themselves in a room in part of the rig, hoping the fire would burn out or emergency systems would kick in.

Eventually three men, realising this wouldn't work, made it to the edge of the platform, and stood staring into one of the world's coldest and roughest oceans. They had two choices – to stay where they were and hope for possible rescue from the flames, or to jump into the freezing ocean and risk almost certain death from hypothermia. Two men chose to jump – and they lived, despite being terribly injured, thanks to a rescue operation mounted by sea. The man who chose to stay put, sadly, perished, as helicopters failed to make it in time.

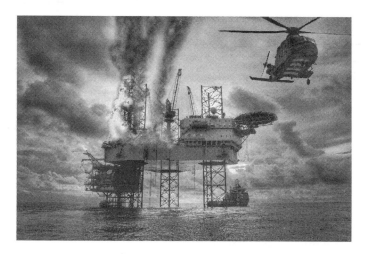

That story contains some powerful learning about the need to respond positively and proactively to serious strategic challenges. It also offers a clue about how to communicate about such challenges.

First, there is the idea of the *unacceptable option of staying the same*. The man who stayed put on the rig in the case study died essentially because he waited for someone else to help him. Staying the same – not going through the change – and hoping things will get better is to risk probable failure.

Second is the message that sometimes *radical, risky change* is *essential*, if painful. Against the odds, the two who jumped survived, though they broke their legs in the process. It hurt, but the action they took gave them the very slight advantage they needed. Above all they took action.

So a burning platform is so serious that it requires action. A burning platform requires a response to an acknowledged crisis, choosing from a limited number of difficult and challenging options. These choices are irreversible and each choice has a high risk of failure.

If we accept that English general practice faces a burning platform situation – and I do – then this book is written to describe a route away from it towards safety. This is not an academic textbook to support research and practice in the sector as this is already well catered for [3]; rather this is a book to support evolution of the sector to ensure it remains fit for purpose as the world around it changes.

At the epicentre of this burning platform, which is the current state of the English primary care sector, are the problems facing current general practitioners and concerns about their future as GPs or family doctors. This book is primarily written for them, from my experience as a GP or family doctor, to offer one vision or description of the future of the primary care sector. That is, being able to put all the evidence together across the primary care sector, which includes changes in their role as GPs or family doctors: from being the omnipotent Dr Finlay type of model practitioner, one who provided all the care he can to his (and it was largely a male preserve) patients, provided the practice premises, employed the staff referred when appropriate to specialist colleagues, and often worked in partnership with one or more other GPs. The GP who worked alongside district nurses and midwives in the local area and other colleagues and clinicians such as mental health and palliative care nurses, pharmacists and counsellors, and social workers and school nurses. From this *traditional model* of the omnipotent GP at the centre of a network of healthcare providers in the community we are moving into a future which GPs and other clinicians can rely on and commit to. We are moving through from the current burning platform of

1. Workload pressures resulting from demographic and clinical practice changes and the increasing burden of complex multi-morbidity and frailty.
2. Workforce problems, with recruitment and retention of clinical staff being particularly problematic for doctors and nurses.
3. Falling practice profitability, where after a decade of austerity, the partners' take-home pay has been in decline.
4. Increasing accountability, with falling popularity and respect from the population alongside a rigorous inspection programme from the Care Quality Commission (CQC), which shines lights into forgotten corners and asks awkward questions before rating each practice and enforcing "quality improvements" across the sector for the first time.
5. At the same time as the key features of general practice, such as the role of the GP as *gatekeeper* to the rest of the NHS, are being challenged by walk-in

centres and hubs, NHS 111, and minor injury units along with new empowered independent practitioners such as advanced nurse practitioners (ANPs), paramedics, clinical pharmacists and physiotherapists – all providing some gatekeeping functions or referral to other parts of the service.

6. *Registration,* another key feature of general practice, which is becoming less relevant and central to the model, as access to online services such as digital provision are emerging as an alternative option for many.

7. Another key feature, *continuity of care,* is increasingly tricky when so many practitioners work part-time, and as a result many locums and salaried clinicians are employed to supplement the self-employed GP partner workforce. Knowledge of people's past medical history is increasingly reliant on comprehensive, reliable, properly coded medical records, rather than on long-term, trust-based relationships between people with good memories. (My first receptionist when I became a GP was Pam or "Aunty Pam" as everyone called her. She knew everyone and all their biographies. She had been the practice receptionist for my predecessor for over twenty years. Without her I would have been lost, and reliable records, while nowhere near as comprehensive as Pam's memory, are essential for continuity of care in a modern service.)

8. Professional partnership has been the dominant business model of general practice since the beginning of the NHS, but is now seen as less attractive to many trained GPs, who see a career as a locum or salaried doctor as meeting their own personal needs and career aspirations without the responsibilities and burdens that they see as requirements of the partnership option.

9. The registered GP has been the holder of the "lifelong" biographical medical record since registration was introduced, but access to the record has become more of an issue as new providers and clinicians (walk in centres and out-of-hours GP services, for example) have emerged requiring access to the information about the people who consult with them. While it remains a key feature of the NHS that the lifelong record is maintained, it does need to inform our care wherever we attend, and currently the somewhat discoordinated sector is not able to ensure that.

10. On the other side of the consultation is an increasingly elderly population with increasingly complex health problems, taking a range of medicines long term, and requiring a level of knowledge skills and experience well beyond that available to previous generations.

It is this multi-legged platform which the book traces the history of. It describes the forces driving the platform towards a future vision which can inspire future generations of clinicians. This is a sector which provides for an increasing proportion of the populations health needs, spanning aspects of social care as well healthcare – covering treatment and prevention of disease, providing cradle-to-grave personal, expert generalist care to the whole population through a system which has the confidence of all parties. The transition from the burning platform involves adapting to a digital future, in the same way that the retail and personal banking sectors are adapting to the digital world by moving their services online. This is a world where access to GPs is no longer dependent on telephone systems;

almost everyone in the community is now able to access data and information online and frequently consult "Dr Google" before they consult their GP. But we are all vulnerable when we are sick, frail, or worried and at these times we need trusted, professional expert advice and care. We need access to services which can address our needs in a timely way, and we need care which respects us as individuals.

Although this transition involves moving away from key historic features of the GP's role, there are some aspects that remain and are vital to the future of the whole provision of healthcare.

1. *The team's diagnostician.* While respecting the contribution of all members of the clinical team, GPs through their training at undergraduate and postgraduate levels have acquired diagnostic skills as expert generalists, which remain as essential now as in the past. Being able to bring all the evidence together from the individual's history, examination and investigations; to accept advice and input from other members of the team; and provide a diagnosis requires considerable expertise based on experience, which GPs are trained to contribute.

2. *Decision making.* We all make decisions every day, but some decisions are trickier and more difficult to make than others. General practitioners, through training and experience, are particularly well equipped to support clinical decision making:
   - By people consulting them who need to make decisions about their health and healthcare both for their present circumstances or for their own future.
   - By the rest of the team – in both clinical situations and for planning the organisation of care.
   - For the organisation. In a GP partnership the responsibility lies with the partners, and unlike consultants in the hospital who have sometimes moved away from "being responsible" as they were when it was their name on the patients bed, in a general practice partnership, partners remain liable – and this can be difficult when partners disagree or are affected by different personal circumstances.

3. *Continuity of care.* While all members of the clinical team are responsible for providing clinical care and will frequently provide continuity during a particular episode of care, GPs, because they often remain in post for long periods of time, are often seen as the link to join up care over time. As more GPs join the rest of the clinical team in working part-time and moving around more frequently than their predecessors did, this continuity is threatened – nevertheless people often remember who their GP is and really value this aspect of their role.

4. *Complex care pathway management.* While much of the clinical work crossing a general practice threshold each day will involve self-limiting conditions or minor complaints, sometimes things can be more complex, particularly as we age and become more frail, so complex multi-morbidity situations arise which require GP skills and experience to help individuals and their families navigate. (*I recently saw a ninety-year-old woman with heart failure in addition*

to her mild dementia. She was in pain from hurting her ribs in a fall. Her carers and her TEP [treatment escalation plan] were clear that hospital admission was not an option.) These kinds of situations are everyday occurrences for GPs – and they learn how to cope "given the circumstances".

This book is also written for all those interested in the future of healthcare, primarily in the UK and primarily outside hospital, but it will draw on international experience and have implications for other sectors of care such as Care provided in hospital and in the social care sector. This book is a journey – it will equip you with the tools to analyse the environment of the primary care sector and this will help you analyse and understand issues you experience within the sector. Although this book is a challenge to the sector, at its heart it is offering a motivating, positive vision for the future of the sector. Those who use the sector, those who work in it, and those who rely on it as the foundation of modern welfare provision in the United Kingdom need this kind of redesign to ensure the sector remains fit for purpose in the digital age. The redesign will inspire you and counter the poor morale, negativism and demotivation that may sell papers and make news, but does a disservice to the really excellent opportunities, the mostly good and outstanding quality of care the sector provides, and the respect and trust which the sector receives from the community it serves.

I come from a background of general practice, born into a family where my father was a rural dispensing doctor and my mother his nurse and only staff member. Our dining room was his consulting room, and my babysitter was the local district nurse, health visitor and midwife (see Box 1.1).

My first work for the health service was to roll up crepe bandages for my father's varicose vein clinic each week and to assemble pillboxes from the flat-packs; aged five, this earned me my pocket money. Some years later, the first local health centre was built over the village pond, and my father's career ended in the 1970s with a stable GP partnership and a well-functioning primary care team. After university and training as a GP, I have spent my entire career working in the sector, primarily as a family doctor but also with experience of *academic* life leading a master's programme; *health service management*; as a primary care trust (PCT) medical director; and *quality assurance and inspection*, as regional adviser and GP specialist adviser for the CQC; and as an assessor for the GMC reviewing the performance of doctors whose performance had been identified as a "cause for concern". I now see patients in the *urgent care* environment through sessional work for the local out-of-hours provider, and support CQC in its programme of regulating the *digital, independent health and primary care sectors*. This book has resulted from the experience wrapped up in this career – the reflections come from the perspective that such a career provides and has been enriched by the experience of the stories I have heard and been part of.

Chapters 2–4 look at the heritage and current performance of the sector – how and why CQC it is delivering mostly "good" or "outstanding" performance [4] – and offer a reflective and critical analysis of the challenges the sector is facing. Although the book's primary focus is on general practice, the issues faced by all the other parts of the primary care sector of the NHS make this analysis just as

BOX 1.1: Joyce's story

Joyce was and had always been a community nurse. After qualifying at St Mary's Paddington, she trained as a midwife, health visitor and district nurse before moving to the Chilterns in 1939. Employed by the county nursing association, she was responsible for the nursing care of a scattered rural community in an area of over 100 square miles. She lived in a tied house, drove an Austin 7 provided for her, had few holidays and little time off. She lived frugally, but was respected and cherished by the local community – free nursing care was available to everyone, even if the doctor had to be paid.

Joyce worked closely with Dr Elliott, the local general practitioner, who lived in a large house with an attached consulting room and dispensary. They frequently used their complementary skills in partnership; they respected and supported each other – but they did not mix socially, did not consult together and were quite clear that doctors' orders were what drove the system.

Early in the World War II, Dr Elliott had a stroke and became less mobile. There was no other medical care available, so Joyce spent much of her time acting as his eyes and ears – doing nearly all the home visiting, acting as his driver and confidant – and developing a healthy respect for his judgement. Three hundred home deliveries were carried out with virtually no backup available, as the flying squad in Oxford was over two hours away. Chronic and acute disease, such as TB, cancer, osteomyelitis and sepsis were dealt with before antibiotics, childhood fevers before immunisation, and pregnancy before scans or rhesus testing.

Following the war, things gradually improved with the arrival of the NHS, more medical and nursing staff, the telephone and television. In the 1960s Joyce married. She had to give up her pension rights, nurse's bungalow and car as those went with the job which was not a married person's post. When she retired, she was feted by the community she had given so much of her life to - so parties and presents but no pension for Joyce.

Twenty years later, widowed and not in the best of health, Joyce was living in a private care home. Her cottage was sold to pay the fees. Her story is told (as she instructed) alongside that of her recent experience in hospital – the noise, the delays, the fog of post-op confusion, and the kindness of ancillary staff and old friends. There is no benevolent fund for Joyce, and she did not want charity; there was no home for retired nurses where she could be among her peers. There were only her wonderful memories, her experience and the love and respect of the community to fortify her and to be talked about whenever I visited her (Rest in peace Joyce who died in 2004).

relevant to them – they all work in partnership with general practice which sits at the centre of the Primary care sector's web. Vignettes and brief case studies are used to illustrate and add colour to the picture and frequently reflect a further vital perspective: that of the people using the sector – patients, citizens, service users or consumers.

Chapters 5–8 uses the tools of *systems thinking* [1] to test the analysis – to challenge the assumptions, question attitudes and make us think differently. These tools are based on research and practice in many different sectors across the world and have proven transformative for organisations ranging from governments and multinational corporations to small businesses and individuals.

Chapters 9 and 10 bring together the results of applying the systems thinking approach to the sector, alongside the analysis of the current performance of the sector and the issues that it is facing. This is reinforced by the results of the CQC inspection programmes in the sector to provide one "vision of the future" to inspire, motivate and provide a direction of travel to the current picture. The transformation that the sector is currently going through is moving it:

- From being a first point of contact, with expert generalist care provided to the whole population through a process of registration and maintenance of a lifelong medical record.
- Towards becoming the entry point for care provided outside hospital, that is, based around the home, for the whole population whether it be in person or using digital technology; providing generalist care over time (biographical) or specialist care when required (episodic) supported by a comprehensive personal healthcare record; and providing both medical and healthcare, social care and community care twenty-four hours a day every day. The care is largely funded from general taxation rather than being privately funded by individual contribution or insurance policy or through co-payment arrangements, where general taxation is "topped-up" by personal contributions which will feature to an extent agreed by the community and which may vary with time.

In order to understand, analyse and critically evaluate any system, it is necessary to explore the following aspects.

- *How the sector has developed.* Its heritage, its responsibilities and its historic relationships: the values, attitudes and beliefs of those who work within the sector and the value of this heritage to the wider public services, the community it serves, and the endowment this heritage provides for future generations.
- *The elements making up the system.* We are taught to analyse problems by breaking them down to their constituent parts; it makes it simpler to understand each element if we can look at it on its own. The only problem is that if we take a machine to pieces completely and understand each element, it may be very difficult to put it back together again. Anyone who has disassembled a car engine or a sewing machine will understand the difficulties. Nevertheless it does make it easier to understand the whole system if we have some appreciation of its constituent parts.

- *Synthesising the elements.* If we are to understand the primary care system, we need to appreciate that each of the elements plays a part in the workings of the whole system. We need to understand the interrelationship of the elements and the part that each plays in maximising the efficiency and effectiveness of the whole. We will look at a number of ways of understanding how the primary care system works so that we have not just an appreciation of the laws or rules governing its behaviour but also sufficient understanding to be able to analyse problems that arise and attempt to devise reasonable solutions to them.
- *What fuels the system?* It is all very well to take an engine to pieces, understand how the elements work, put it back together again, see how all the elements interact with each other and what the purpose of each element is, etc., but we also need to understand what powers the engine. Any system requires energy or resources to drive it, and the primary care system is no different. As well as requiring energy as an input, the system will also produce energy as an output. While a car engine turns petrol into the force to make the car travel down the road, the primary care system uses human resources and money to provide care for the population. After a decade of austerity, where the input of resources, after allowing for inflation, demographic change and rising infrastructure costs has failed to grow at all, there have been understandably strident cries for more resources, understandable promises from the taxpayer for jam tomorrow and increasing difficulty in recruiting people whose take-home pay is dependent on the bottom line or the profitability of their business. Car manufacturers, faced with similar issues as a result of global oil prices, have made more efficient engines and looked to alternative fuels, such as electricity. The primary care system similarly will need to look beyond the taxpayer if it is to maintain its power output; it will need to reform the way it operates, integrate care by melting barriers, and develop business models which are more efficient by design, greener and more sustainable by culture, and as a result are more resilient.

Understanding its heritage and analysing the primary care system can help us to interpret how fit the sector is for its current and developing responsibilities. Using the tools of systems thinking [1] should help us to see not only the wood for the trees but also the wood and the trees.

Whether you are a professional practitioner in the sector, a student of health policy, an interested citizen using the sector to obtain advice and treatment for a health problem, or a director of a corporate organisation providing healthcare in the sector, you will already have relevant knowledge and experience which will help you appreciate this book and understand how to use the tools it describes so that together they can help you become master of your primary healthcare.

After almost seventy years, the NHS is facing major challenges. The complexity and costs of modern health services and the needs of the society within which those services are provided have changed dramatically since the early post-war years when those services were designed. That design may have been fit for purpose in 1947 and the services may have evolved through a whole series of redesigns – or tinkerings – over the years, but the fundamental design features have remained the same, and perhaps this is unique in this country where little from the 1940s has escaped radical transformation in the intervening years. (See reference [5] – the foundation of the NHS.)

This book will help you analyse the current challenges the NHS is facing, particularly in the primary care sector, and help you answer the question of whether the service remains fit for purpose. While modern general practices still have Lloyd George envelopes (our legacy from the 1910s) containing our paper health records, stored away and brought out to complete insurance reports or transfer to another practice when we move around the country, they are a link to the past. I remember writing in them in the early 1980s and using them to construct people's medical histories when introducing computer systems into practice in the early 1990s. But they are not the major repository of our medical history; that is now held online, and unlike too many acute hospital records, they are usually fit to underpin the provision of safe, high-quality, efficient and effective healthcare. Now we need to transform the holder of those records, the provider of healthcare through the use of those records, into an organisation and sector that is similarly a safe, high-quality, efficient and effective provider.

As new technology allows more care to be provided while we continue to live at home, then a greater proportion of health resources will be used there. As the population ages and as everyone expects better health and healthcare, so the responsibilities of those providing home-based care increase and the providers of care will need to be proportionately more accountable for their use of resources and the quality of care they are providing. The changing dynamics of the whole system resulting from primary care have the responsibility

- To *commission* hospital-based care (through clinical commissioning groups).
- To *Assess* the health needs of the local community (in partnership with public health).
- To work in *partnership* with local authority social services.

This still places primary care at the centre of the NHS. Now it requires a sector design which is fit to help it meet these responsibilities in a modern, digital world. If we are to access TV and radio in a bespoke "personal fashion" rather than the set menu offered in the radio and TV times, then we have to consider whether our access to personal welfare services – health and social care – requires similar rethinking.

We cannot continue to rely on historic constructs such as the concept of "partnership" or the ideal of "integrated care" or a "local health economy" to provide rather vague, ill-defined solutions to all the system's problems. Analysing and strengthening what partnership working means should help us develop a range of organisational arrangements which suit the needs of the local population. On the whole, relationships and systems work the way they do because that is how they have been designed and evolved to work. The primary care sector needs and deserves a redesign to ensure it remains fit for the future.

This then is the agenda. The book does not seek to impart facts, but rather to help you construct, understand, analyse and criticise. Above all, the book seeks to liberate your own thinking so that you can grasp the opportunity to transform home-based care.

INTERNATIONAL PERSPECTIVES

A small group was invited to address some key questions from their own experience. The group was drawn from the UK, Europe, New Zealand, Australia, the United States and Canada. Their comments are as biased as my own, but do help to provide some balance to the narrative. By and large they reflect that all our populations and their health providers face similar issues which are stressing our health systems. Some lessons from abroad have informed this analysis and suggestions that the later chapters contain.

Questions for the international panel

Questions for the international commentators to consider and respond to:

1. A key feature of my experience in England is its *workforce crisis* – not enough GPs – promises to recruit more but people retiring early, working part-time and migrating abroad. Locum usage and costs are rocketing. More nurses, pharmacists, physios and counsellors working in the sector but reluctant to take responsibility. *How is it where you are?*
2. England is experiencing *demographic pressure* from the frail elderly, often with complex multi-morbidity issues complicated by social isolation and the difference between personal payment for social care as against the "free" NHS is often problematic. *How is it where you are?*
3. Pressure on *profitability* following a decade of austerity has affected English general practice, retail pharmacy and pay across the whole sector, and although the NHS long-term plan is promising more cash, we are still waiting. In addition the contracting arrangements, employment and tax status of staff, access to capital for premises and the effect of the "inverse care law" are having perverse effects on plans to improve health and healthcare. *How are you tackling these issues and what can you teach us?*
4. Increased demand, from the worried well and those with minor illness, is a feature in England affecting general practice and the urgent care sector. While many have expanded their capacity, too many are still drowning in demand. *How are things where you are?*
5. Registration, the lifelong record held by the GP, expert generalism, continuity of care and funding through general taxation have been key features of the NHS primary care system. Some of them are being questioned by current pressures in England. *Does the different context and environment where you are mean that you are responding to pressure in different ways?*
6. While the pre-eminence of the "medical model" in the primary care sector remains largely unquestioned, the biopsychosocial, social and green agendas have altered some of the power dynamics underpinning modern medicine's position in English general practice. *To what extent is medicine still the dominant player in your primary care system?*

7. My book points towards a sector where "active citizenship" and "empowered patients" (responsible for their own lifelong record for example), mutuality (communitarianism) and redefined professionalism (advisers and teachers rather than omnipotent) are characteristics. *How does that feel from your perspective?*

8. Coordination of care across organisational boundaries has long been difficult within the NHS, and despite progress with information technology systems there remain problems between primary and secondary care, between the NHS and other care providers such as social services, and between different parts of the primary care sector such as general practice and the urgent care sector providers. *What can the NHS in England learn from your experience?*

9. As we move into an increasingly digital world with retail, banking, education and much commercial business moving online: *What should the NHS be doing to develop a digital offering to the population? What has happened where you are and is any of it transferable?*

10. *What do you feel the healthcare system where you are should learn from the NHS in England?*

Their responses

1. *Workforce crisis.* Following a survey of its membership, the Royal College of General Practitioners (RCGP) Scotland [6] published its findings about the state of general practice in Scotland in eight chapters with thirty associated recommendations and areas for further action. The report mirrors many of the same features as found in my experience of English general practice, but Scotland's experience of deprivation, rurality, variation in life expectancy, and different experience of morbidity as a result of drug and alcohol dependency (particularly opiate abuse) have all meant extra stress on Scottish General practice.

   In Wales and Northern Ireland, similar issues are highlighted: workforce problems and changing demography, exacerbated where there are social and rural deprivation, are features of practice, placing additional demands on an overstretched workforce. In fact, the underlying issues are global [7], as Roy Lilley points out. New York is facing difficulty recruiting clinicians, a rising tide of the frail elderly with complex medical problems, and apart from fitting air-conditioning units in care homes (to reduce emergency hospital admissions during hot spells) it is still searching for answers. New Zealand, Australia and Canada report similar, if nascent, workforce problems with 70% of New Zealand GPs saying they are working in a practice with a current GP vacancy or had had one in the past year. The numbers of nurse practitioners are increasing to help fill the gap.

2. *Demographic pressures.* From the rising number of the elderly, often with complex health problems, are not restricted to England. All countries responding report multi-morbidity as an issue. This is particularly the case in New Zealand and Australia among Maoris and other "ethnic populations"

and by people living socially isolated lives. In Wales, rural isolation adds an additional pressure.

3. *Profitability.* Inevitably, responses here are specific to the predominant business model in the country, but in the UK where professional partnership predominates, the issue of Partnership profitability being under pressure is reported from everywhere. Because practices, like all professional partnerships, do not publish their accounts, there remains no clarity on the extent of this pressure and how it varies across the UK. But it is inevitably a factor in determining whether doctors decide to become profit-sharing partners whose take home pay is directly related to the profitability and adversely affected by declining profitability. In countries where *co-payment* by individual patients as well as by government is a key feature, such as New Zealand, Australia and parts of Europe, then there is a consensus that profitability is under pressure, whereas in countries where market forces and insurance cover are more predominant, costs are increasing and providers are reporting pressure on profits but are able to raise their charges to compensate.

4. *Drowning in demand.* Across the UK, all general practice respondents report similar issues with "inappropriate demand" affecting practices' ability to cope, and have been introducing triage and "alternative clinician approaches" (particularly ANPs) in response. Co-payment systems seem to help to reduce this tendency, but they are also introducing "filtration systems" to manage increasing demand (triage systems of one type or another). There is a common feeling that emergency department (ED) services being free at the point of care encourages inappropriate attendance, but data suggests that while some of the ED volume is low acuity in nature, most of the growth is in those with high acuity issues (New Zealand).

5. *The influence of key features.* All respondents concur with the English experience of pressure on the key features leading to *continuity of care place* rather than continuity of practitioner. Continuity, shared records and expert generalism are moving GPs and their practices towards "community complex care specialism". Moves away from taxation funding towards a more US style of free market funding are not supported by respondents who all remain committed to *whole population coverage* as a key feature. The issues raised by registration, as a key characteristic of the NHS, were not focussed on by respondents. But membership of or coverage by insurance is an important feature of all places where the private sector rather than the state is the commissioner.

6. *The medical model.* The medical model remains predominant everywhere. Although moves towards multi-professional team working are common features, the dominance and power remain in medical hands. Commentators also point out that patient empowerment and stronger roles for pharmacy, psychological therapists, midwives and nursing have affected the power dynamic of the "medical model", and certainly alternative medicine and the impact of the third sector are influential in some situations, for example the success of immunisation programmes. Nevertheless, in all the responding countries, the power – coming from knowledge, acknowledged expertise, control of resources and decision making – remain mainly in doctors hands.

7. *Active citizenship and empowered patients.* These are common themes across the responders but to varying degrees. Co-payment is seen as empowering in New Zealand and Australia, as is "ownership" of the clinical record, but while "many would sign up to the vision they recognise that years of professional custom and practice need to be transformed to enable any true shift of power" (New Zealand). Moves towards a common record, or shared access to records, is another common theme, Welsh individual health records (IHRs) and English summary care records for example. These do improve care coordination, as do shared access to results and electronic referral systems, but these are all seen as *incremental* and *adaptive* approaches to improving care rather than any systematic *transformative* answer to the common problem in all the systems responding: the lack of care integration or *truly shared care.*

8. *Care coordination.* The weakness of this is discussed earlier, but the Australian electronic system "My Health Record" is regarded as useful, despite the omission of social care providers, the voluntary sector and allied health providers from the team of contributors and users. Responders all support moves towards better care coordination but apart from "My health record" in Australia have no other initiatives to offer the NHS in England.

9. *Digital offering.* The situation seems to be similar to England. Some interest in Skype consulting in Wales, support of isolated practice and practitioners may be a factor, and the use of texting and "My Health Online" is also popular in some arenas. Access to a patient portal for GPs and patients seems to be popular in New Zealand and there is also support for a new digital platform to coordinate care there, which has a strong history in being early adopters of digital technology to support care pathway redesign. There are emerging challenges from multiple platforms developing and working in isolation and sometimes without coordination by primary care. While it is recognised that a digital healthcare offering is required in the world we all live in, none of the respondents offer examples of what it needs to look like. Respondents from British-based digital healthcare providers (those I have visited and been involved with regulating through the Care Quality Commission) have mostly been targeting either medicine supplies or have a segmented approach to consultation with particular subsets of the population, mostly working-age people with acute health concerns. Moving from this segmented approach to a more holistic offer – from preconceptual counselling to supporting grief and bereavement – and offering the package to the whole population is acknowledged as an aspiration, but not realistic or deliverable at present.

10. *Learning from the NHS in England.* "Free care at the point of need" is a big issue for countries where people have to pay upfront for care, in the United States and Australia for example but also in many European countries. New Zealand responses emphasise the importance of following England by investing in a strong primary care sector, but caution against using structural change as a solution to system problems and also mention the difficulty of moving monolithic structures and the problem of "traditionalist" thinking. In Australia, access to specialist care is difficult and expensive and, as in the United States, the uninsured are excluded from care.

With particular thanks to Dr Helen Parker (New Zealand), Prof Tony Dowell (New Zealand), Dr Mark Thomas (Wales), Dr Carey Lunan (Scotland) and Dr Andrew Roxburgh (Australia).

REFLECTION: SOCIAL CARE AND HEALTHCARE – BOTH PARTS OF THE WELFARE SYSTEM

The demise of the generic, practice-attached, local authority social worker following reforms in the 1970s caused me a couple of problems, and this will have been mirrored across the country. Margaret P was a force of nature – revered and feared in equal measure in our small town – but with a vocation to protect anyone who fell off the ladder. JT, my predecessor as local GP, had died suddenly while cycling back from his boat, and Margaret came to see me. "I need to take you to see two people who JT knew about and should now become your responsibility". First was Catherine. She was in her thirties and unknown to the authorities other than Margaret and JT, who had not been allowed to intervene. Catherine was the product of incest and was cared for by her mother, aunt and uncle, all now becoming elderly. I knew the aunt, having recently referred her to get her cataracts dealt with, while her mother had mild learning disabilities and her uncle was going to need a hip operation soon. Catherine was naked and lying in a large cot in the living room of their prefab bungalow. She was blind and had no speech, she was fitting and had a spastic quadriplegia.

Next, Margaret took me to see David. We went to a clearing in local scrub woodland where in a small hut David lay "in extremis". He had been a local tramp for some years; locals remembered him selling clothes pegs, doing odd jobs and moving on before the local police arrived. Now he looked very ill and had asked Margaret to summon help from the NHS; he'd paid for it during the war but never registered or used it. After assessment under the powers of the National Assistance Act and with the help of the local public health consultant, he ended up receiving palliative care in a local care home, where he died a couple of weeks later from what turned out to be tertiary syphilis.

Amidst the social revolution of recent years – and now the digital revolution – the demise of the heritage that Margaret represented has its consequences everywhere. People like Catherine and David are part of every community. We all see the homeless begging in the street every day and are all too familiar with the stories of serious case reviews such as that into the death of Victoria Columbie and the horrifying case of Dr Harold Shipman, but I would reflect that the failure of *responsibility* this represents may be the price we have to pay for our personal freedoms, but it is a heavy price.

REFERENCES

1. Senge PM. 1990. *The Fifth Discipline*. Currency and Doubleday, New York.
2. Washington M. 2011. *Successful Organisational Transformation*. Business Expert Press, New York.

3. Greenhalgh T. 2007. *Primary Health Care Theory and Practice*. Blackwell Press, Malden, MA.
4. Care Quality Commission (CQC). 2017. The state of care in general practice 2014 to 2017.
5. Ministry of Health. 1946. *National Health Services Bill*. Summary of the proposed new service. CMD 6761. HMSO, London.
6. Royal College of General Practitioners Scotland. 2019. From the frontline: The changing practice of Scottish general practice.
7. Lilley R. 2019. Do the right thing [blog]. NHS Managers.net. 21 October.

2

Keystones

1. What has constituted the primary care sector? *What have been the defining characteristics?*
2. What does the concept of *sustainability* mean within the sector?
3. What does the concept of *resilience* imply in the sector?
4. How can we ensure that the sector is *trustworthy*?

I provide a few reflections on how the system copes with these key issues. Each of these key issues (keystones) requires consideration from a range of perspectives: that of the individual (both those working in the sector and those who use its services), the teams responsible for providing care, the organisations responsible for providing care, and of the sector as a whole.

DEFINING CHARACTERISTICS

For the sake of clarity, the primary care sector has received many definitions over the years. Barbara Starfield's 1994 [1] approach has received widespread support: "The level of a Healthcare system that provides entry into the system for all needs and problems, it provides person-focussed – rather than disease-oriented care, care over time, providing care for all but vey uncommon or unusual conditions, and coordinates or integrates care provided elsewhere by others". Accepted characteristics in the UK primary care systems include:

- First point of contact care. The place where every citizen goes first to access care: the chemist shop for medicines; the optician for eye care, glasses and contact lenses; and the general medical practice for healthcare, prevention of disease, medical and nursing treatment, referral and support.
- A holistic approach. A broad approach considering the individual's health needs in the context of their psychological and emotional state, their life situation and their lifestyle, their past and current health problems and issues, and their life aspirations and plans.
- Care to a registered, undifferentiated population, unsegmented by age, gender, ethnicity, current health status or future health risk profile.

- Continuing responsibility for care over time. Joining the individual on their journey rather than just seeing them through an episode of care. In recent times a greater range of specialist care is being provided in the primary care sector and a greater range of providers have emerged who do not always restrict care to a registered population (e.g. walk-in centres, out-of-hours providers, triage services [NHS 111, for example]). While general practitioners remain sensitive about their heritage and status ([2] the truth is that their future is as a vital part of the primary care sector where their medical expertise as expert generalists is vital to the population and to the efficiency and effectiveness of the whole primary care sector. Given the emerging realignment of care provision promoted by technical and demographic change, it may well be that previous definitions and sector divisions need to be reviewed. The challenge is to consider the out of hospital provision of health and social care in a digital world where health outcomes and the processes through which they are achieved are more important than the structures or organisations through which they are delivered rather than an updated version of a traditional general practice or a narrow consideration of medical care. The requirement is to consider the individual's health and welfare and deliver it using expert generalist medical alongside other services in the sector such as specialist medical support provided as outreach from hospital services, nursing care of all types, community pharmacy services, optician services and all interventions working alongside individual citizens as their life unfolds, supported by the expertise of a range of associated professions and workers, including some whose role in the sector is currently marginal but needs to be consolidated and their value enhanced such as

  * Palliative care nurses and their teams,
  * Community mental health practitioners and their teams,
  * Learning disability teams,
  * Community nursing teams – both generalist and specialist,
  * Midwives and health visitors,
  * Counsellors social workers and their teams.

This is irrespective of their current employment status – if their professional work and careers are within the Primary care sector then they need to be considered as integral parts of the sector as do people living and working in the nursing and residential care home sector and those in supported independent living units in the community. They have important health and welfare needs and are frequent users of the sector and contribute to the stresses it faces.

These stresses and their implications are discussed in later chapters and the tools to understand their impact are described.

SUSTAINABILITY

With over ninety percent of patient contacts with the National Health Service (NHS) happening in the primary care sector, concerns about sustainability matter to all of us and have implications to all the other sectors that care for the population.

Many individuals in the workforce have a lack of confidence in their future – they sometimes feel that their role is unsustainable – either because of high workload or lack of support or lack of confidence in the future course they perceive as being set. The recent workforce survey among GPs in the South West of England [3] illustrates this: "A substantial majority of GPs in South West England report low morale. Many are considering career intentions which, if implemented, would adversely impact GP workforce capacity within a short time period". The issue is not confined to GPs; the nursing workforce is also affected and with clinicians concerned about the sustainability of their role the rest of the workforce is inevitably caught up in the cultural backlash.

Local people, users of the service, also have emerging concerns about sustainability [4]. Feedback from user groups, both online and through filtration via representative groups or the Care Quality Commission [5] inspection programme, shows that stressed access arrangements, lack of continuity of care and confusion about how to use services appropriately is widespread. While there is a continuing high level of confidence in "my local service", user uncertainty is leading to inappropriate behaviour. Rising numbers ending up in accident and emergency (A&E), walk-in centres and hubs being used for routine rather than urgent care and GP surgeries being drowned in the care of people with acute, often self-limiting sickness rather than addressing the long-term care needs of their population – including those with long-term conditions such as diabetes, cancer, learning disabilities and multiple sclerosis – are another example of the *inverse care law* [7] where the demands of those with least needs prevent resources reaching those with the greatest needs. To have confidence in a sustainable future for the sector, users need to believe that the sector and the NHS will be there for them when they need it, that their care is safe in its hands, that their care will be coordinated efficiently, and that their needs and views will be respected.

What about the sustainability of the primary care team? In the past, general practitioners and their employed staff worked closely with local community staff (district nurses, midwives, health visitors, specialist palliative care nurses, etc.) and social care professionals from the local authority to form a "team". Although the team consisted of a group of clinicians working together despite organisational and cultural boundaries and without any coherent, agreed plan of activity – beyond supporting each other to respond to individual caseload and agreed action plans – in many places it worked effectively. The team has been in decline for some years, as initiatives such as community nursing teams, patch health visiting in response to the development of children's centres, generic social workers, and the destabilising effect of organisational turbulence, where nurses in particular have had multiple employers, have emerged. As a result, the recent CQC inspection programme [6] in the sector has found the effective primary care team to be the exception rather than the rule, with consequent lack of effectiveness in the delivery of care. For example vulnerable children, mothers with young babies, the frail elderly and those with dementia – those whose needs are greatest – are being denied evidence-based, effective, coordinated care. Despite good and outstanding practices and best efforts to coordinate care, their success and high-quality patient care is *despite their difficulties rather than because of their strengths*. No wonder many clinicians feel that the sustainability of the primary care team is far from assured. The historic definition of the primary care team this refers to requires transformation. To transform current almost vestigial primary care healthcare teams and drive effective and efficient care through them requires revision of policy and practise, protocols and procedures; shared priorities and training; empowerment and enfranchisement of these new teams. Not just a call for more resources, just a call for realignment and new thinking – glasnost and perestroika (they knocked down the Berlin Wall) – which can transform teams and team working, encompassing new professions and workers all brought together to work as teams because they add value as team members rather than providers of isolated services – part of becoming an orchestra rather than a group of soloists.

How sustainable are the organisations providing care in the sector?

Other chapters will consider the future of primary care provider organisations in more detail; here we will simply address the question of sustainability. To ensure organisational sustainability requires a belief among those responsible for the organisations that their investment in finance, energy, time and commitment is safe; that there is agreement with partner organisations about their plans and their priorities; that they will be able grow within a framework where their responsibilities are defined; and that they are held to account for their performance, respected for their expertise and rewarded accordingly (a strong governance framework covering clinical, organisational, corporate and information elements). At present, the array of organisations operating in the sector have faith in the sector but little belief that their faith is sustainable, so their commitment is limited, their investment constrained and their focus relatively short term. The result is GP partnerships in transition to "federations", corporate organisations "supporting" practices or rescuing failing services within short-term contracting arrangements, community interest organisations and social enterprises thriving through the personal commitment of those involved rather than through any coherent governance framework which assures all parties that their faith is justified. This situation is underpinned and the sector's direction set by the NHS "Five Year Forward View" (2015) and its associated papers relating to the sector, but there is a lack of confidence that those responsible will be able to deliver. History tells us, and many primary care organisations believe, that other sectors such as hospitals have louder voices and more power, but they provide a relatively small proportion of care and should not be permitted to dominate thinking and focus in the way they have historically. The following chapters will explore how, in the modern world, more care can be provided in the primary care sector, but organisations need some certainty beyond the "Five Year Forward View" that their future is assured before sustainable organisations can develop.

For the primary care sector to be sustainable it requires some *redefining* to fit within a National Health Service and wider welfare system which confidently describes the relationship between the individual citizen's responsibility for their own health, and the responsibility of government as discharged through local government and the NHS. To ensure the sustainability of the sector it requires its responsibilities to be agreed and resourced rather than care being *transferred* into it by stressed hospitals or shifted around it by lack of social care funding. While the sector cannot be micromanaged as it is currently organised, there is a need for a more joined up approach to its management, so that care coordination is promoted within the sector and the wider NHS and social care sectors, and inefficient duplication of services is curtailed. While the individual citizen's freedom of choice matters, it cannot be allowed to prevent the emergence of a more effective and efficient primary care sector. At present there is a lack of confidence among individuals, teams and organisations within the sector that those with responsibility for commissioning care have the understanding and powers necessary to deliver that more effective and efficient, coordinated care that is required. The history of national contracts driven by history rather than health needs, national negotiating by teams and organisations determined to preserve their own power rather than address the needs of a modern society, provide only short-term fixes to long-term problems – these are a threat to the sustainability of a sector which cannot be allowed to continue. Rather the population requires a sector designed to meet the changing needs of society, within a framework of governance which promotes confidence and is coherent with other partner sectors.

How can we make the sector more sustainable?

Given the various meanings of sustainability we need to be clear that we are not considering the effect of the primary care sector on the environment and whether its use of resources has a positive or negative impact on the planet. We may think that the sector has considerably less impact than the alternatives, where hospital–institutional care is probably more resource intensive and "self care" where the impact on the planet may be less, but the evidence is lacking and the consequences of ineffective care and untreated disease may be much more expensive.

Rather, we are considering the long-term sustainability of the primary care sector and in particular the sustainability of the provision of high-quality, safe care for the population and the sustainability of the workforce providing that care as well as the business models around which the organisations providing care within the sector are formed. While the evidence about these is emerging and quite weak, there is concern about pockets of poor quality, unsafe care within the sector and about poor recruitment and retention of general practitioners and in particular of GP partners, and the future of the various business models underpinning the sector [3]. These elements are considered in more detail in later chapters; here it is sufficient just to comment that we have a sector providing a service of great importance – highly regarded by the population, with a really positive heritage and reputation, which is struggling to sustain high-quality, safe care through current business models, and to maintain a stable workforce in the face of the stresses the sector currently faces.

RESILIENCE

This has been defined in various ways as "maintaining health despite adversity" or "a dynamic, evolving process of positive attitudes and effective strategies" or "the inverted score on a burnout inventory" or to include features such as positive adaptation, development of personal resources, personal growth or a sort of hardiness [5].

How can we promote resilience?

I include all those whose professional work is performed outside hospital – mental health practitioners and their teams, learning disability teams, community nursing teams (both generalists and specialists), midwives and health visitors, counsellors and social workers and their teams, school nurses, staff working for care agencies both in residential care homes and those involved with domiciliary care. This is irrespective of their current employment status; if their professional work is within the sector then they need to be considered as integral parts of that sector. People living in nursing and residential care homes or in supported independent living units in the community have important health and welfare needs and are frequent users of the sector. The training and support and practice of all involved in these locations needs to be brought together to enhance their roles and quality assure their practice.

With the emergence of digital services in recent years we need to be clear that these key characteristics of the sector apply whether citizens are accessing care in person or using digital technology. Providers of digital services need to be regulated and designed to provide the services the population needs rather than feel they can "cherry-pick" to provide episodic care to selected minorities in the community. Currently these digital providers, such as Babylon GP at Hand, are particularly attracting the working age population (see CQC reports on these and other digital providers), but this needs to change, and traditional face-to-face providers need to develop a digital offering or develop partnerships with digital providers to offer digital services to the NHS population.

In this section, I will look at resilience at the individual, team, organisation and sector levels, and the description of resilience as being *a dynamic process encompassing positive adaptation within the context of significant adversity* [5] seems most appropriate.

Individual residence among primary healthcare professionals has been shown to be multifaceted (incorporating individual traits with social and workplace factors), and to be negatively associated with overuse of alcohol, having additional responsibilities such as childcare and running a home, and lack of control over working hours, and positively associated with control of work volume and organisation, personality features such as being highly self directed, accepting of uncertainty, and a sense of purpose or vocation. In addition, lifestyle factors can influence resilience, such as family support, physical exercise and leisure time [5,8].

For the *individual* working in the primary care sector – be they doctor, nurse or other clinician, manager or reception/admin – the forces and factors promoting or reducing resilience are the same. As demand on the sector increases, as the complexity of the work increases and as individuals have less control over their work, less sense of self-value and less feeling of being valued in their team and organisation, their ability to bounce back is reduced.

Strategies to promote individual resilience are needed if the issues of recruitment and retention [3] are to be countered. Although short-term measures like funding for sabbaticals, skill substitution to rearrange workflow, and support groups and federations matter, what is required is a more systematic and planned approach to redefining and supporting every individual working in the sector. Governance arrangements to link individual performance to organisational performance, to support career development and advancement, to provide mentorship and support for counselling and reflection are options. Unless the NHS starts to value the primary care workforce more, then experience shows that a crisis in recruitment and retention of staff in the sector is inevitable. Being self-employed (as GP partners, general dental practitioner partners and independent pharmacists) but contracted to be responsible for NHS patients, to provide NHS care, to employ staff with NHS rights should mean that the NHS has a responsibility to ensure that the GP workforce as well as all of those working in the sector are supported and valued so as to promote individual resilience. This programme might include training, mentoring, personal development support, mindfulness and other psychological programmes, nutrition, exercise and lifestyle advice and support, alongside easy access to rescue support as and when it is needed.

The resilient primary care *team* will need a rescue package if it is to be *reinforced*, because in many places it has become largely rhetorical and symbolic rather than an effective care-providing and coordinating agent. The resilient team will also require a sustained programme of support, including an approach to team governance which can assure users and members that the team is trustworthy, a theme developed further in later chapters. Organisational governance from all the employing organisations has become too dominant. The team has its own rights and responsibilities which have been undervalued for too long. Supporting the team's autonomy and managing it against the team's priorities and key performance indicators is long overdue. Consider how important this is for palliative care, neonatal care and care of those with learning disabilities.

The resilient primary care *organisation*, no matter how it is constituted and commissioned, has the responsibility to provide NHS care to the people using it, and will be assessed by CQC and rated against agreed national standards and criteria. How the organisation is able to bounce back from challenges will be governed by a few key considerations:

- Whether the organisation is *designed* to promote the provision of high-quality, safe, effective and responsive care and demonstrate high-quality leadership.
- Whether the organisation *learns* from and responds to a challenge in such a way as to reduce the impact of further challenges.
- Whether the organisation invests in appropriate *support* to ensure it understands, addresses and reflects on challenges.
- How well the organisation is *integrated* into the rest of the local sector and wider health and welfare economy.

- The extent to which the organisation values and is valued by the local community. To be resilient the organisation will need the support of that community in tough times, and resilience needs to include the concept of mutual support or interdependence. The essential feature is being *open* rather than closed. For too long primary care provider organisations have not been open to public scrutiny, open to community challenge and open to criticism. Governance arrangements have not been helpful and the result is isolation leading to a lack of resilience. As the environment within which the organisations exist changes, they need to adapt if they are to survive.

The primary care sector is also facing challenges and will need to respond [9]. The challenges it faces are the subject of this book. Here it is sufficient just to point out that currently, responsibility for managing, commissioning and regulating the sector, *as a whole*, is unassigned. The responsibility for managing and commissioning is split between NHS England (NHSE), local government, clinical commissioning groups (CCGs) and the third sector. Provider organisations are regulated by the CQC, which has no power to address issues it finds. NHS improvement has no remit within the sector and this gap is a fundamental issue and weakness. The autonomy of the sector where it is alone responsible for the quality of care it provides requires attention. This is different from secondary care or social care where responsible organisations are more clearly defined. As more specialist care is provided in the community, as the schism between health and social care becomes increasingly bad for people's health and well-being, and as technology changes the ground rules (so being stuck with the 1980s definition "first point of contact", etc. [1], seems less sustainable), the distinction would now seem to be between *institutional (hospital for example) or individual-*based care – home based or provided, directed and focussed on the needs of individual people for healthcare or welfare services. To become a resilient sector, *individual-focussed* care needs to reflect on the *SOLID (supported, open, learning, integrated, designed)* considerations introduced earlier and considered further in later chapters.

TRUST

How can we ensure that the sector is trustworthy?

This in essence was the question underlying the original book [7] and it remains central. However, the answer now has additional dimensions. Originally I considered this from the perspective of the individual:

- What makes it safe for me to trust my career to the sector? For a clinician this really means "Does the *clinical governance* framework give me confidence that it is safe for me to commit to the sector?" given the recruitment and retention difficulties and the findings of the CQC inspection programme, many clinicians are uncertain about the answer. By the end of the book I will have offered a prescription or vision to address this.

- What makes it safe for me as a citizen to trust the sector? Surveys continue to show that the GP, general practice and the sector as a whole have maintained high satisfaction among the public, but this has shown recent decline [3]. As society has changed and the design of the sector has adapted, there is less confidence among the younger generation in the traditional general practice, less confidence in the out-of-hours arrangements and the CQC inspection programme, which has been worrying – and far from isolated concerns about arrangements for accessing care, with telephone system problems being a leading concern. If people have concerns about accessing care, then they may well lose the confidence to seek care, particularly if they are insecure, vulnerable, frightened or experiencing mental health or emotional difficulties. High survey performance, like an overall *good performance* in the CQC programme should not be allowed to inspire too much confidence; the headlines may obscure the fault lines.

However, the new dimensions such as those described earlier concerning *sustainability* and *resilience*, along with considerations such as professionalism, assurance, and effective clinical and performance management have to be considered to ensure trustworthiness, not just from the individual's perspective but also from the community's. The funder of the sector is predominantly the taxpayer, either through general taxation or through a variety of top-up arrangements. When the funder has concerns, as described by the House of Commons Select Committee's inquiry into the sector [11], then it calls into question the trustworthiness of the sector and the arrangements through which it assures the community that it is trustworthy.

Keystones and how the system copes

1. Tony – an old friend told me his story: He had been with his GP for over fifty years. His whole family were registered there and he would fly back to the UK to consult there. Thirty years ago he had a serious neurological disease which took him a couple of years to get over and left home with a foot drop when he was tired. His daughter-in-law had died from a rare cancer after several years of highly specialist treatment and other family members had also received ongoing supportive treatment. Tony told me, in the year before he died, that one of the things that made him most proud to be British was that the design of the NHS had supported him and his family to receive ongoing care and treatment. "It has been my security blanket".
2. Angela – a work colleague: "From my point of view the greatest tragedy has been the way the team who cared for my mother in the five years after her stroke has been dissipated and is not there to support her as she copes with her daughter with cystic fibrosis [CF]. The health visitor and district nurse are no longer based in the surgery, the practice team are all part-time and even the reception team don't know me and my issues. I get great specialist support from the tertiary specialist centre and their outreach nurses but they don't seem to work with our GP and her care is really not as joined up as my mum's was. My mum's social worker was a rock when she had to adapt her

home and when she went into a care home – but now support for adaptations for her daughter has been organised through the CF association and the Citizens Advice Bureau and has taken over two years to complete". "Nobody seems to see the whole picture, things are really discoordinated".

3. Rod – a GP colleague told me that the Priory Avenue Practice had been a good practice for many years and a reliable neighbour to his own practice. Then, within a couple of years things went downhill – the four GP partners retired and could not recruit new GPs, the practice manager struggled on with a succession of locum GPs and a practice nurse who knew everyone and had been there for over twenty years. Patient services began to decline and the patients were increasingly unhappy. The local secretary of the LMC tried to offer support, but neither the CCG or the NHSE team could offer any help. An "Inadequate" CQC rating and a spell in "special measures" only led to "support" from a "corporate provider" for a year or two. Now the practice is inching towards a merger with another local practice, but there has been no effective management intervention to enhance resilience. Rather those who commission services from the practice have mimicked Dr Werner von Braun once the rockets are up, who cares where they come down [10].

4. "For me, it all comes down to trust", said Mary. "I have always trusted my GP and the local practice, and I've been with them for over twenty years – but not any more. Last year I needed to see them because I developed a nasty kidney infection – but there were no appointments for over a week. I went to the local 'walk-in' centre and thence to be an emergency admission at the local hospital. I think the GP and practice let me down and I won't trust them again. I'll go to the urgent care sector or the hospital". "Trust is a fragile flower, it takes years to nurture but can disappear over a single incident".

5. Pete had had a nasty bout of encephalitis and been in the local hospital, severely disabled for weeks. He had been referred to a specialist rehab unit sixty miles away but the wait for a bed seemed interminable, so he came home. Services at home were restricted to a physio visiting him weekly for thirty minutes, but his mobility and independence were really poor. Mary, his wife, struggled on. But Pete was losing his confidence and Mary was struggling to cope. A local personal trainer/Pilates teacher (Jane) got involved as a neighbour and really transformed the situation. Over a period of weeks Pete's outlook was transformed; Jane motivated him and Mary. Once they believed he could get better and started actively engaging, he managed to get out of his chair and start walking. Within a few weeks he was able to get out to the pub and then be assessed to drive an automatic car. Within a few months Pete and Mary were off on a holiday by air to Spain, and he was so pleased. The point was that his own empowerment was legitimised by Jane, who then encouraged him to mobilise and get his own life back. Pete trusted Mary and came to trust Jane. I firmly believe that this story could be repeated countless times – there is a place for expert input – but empowerment and motivation, and input from family, neighbours and the local community can make a huge difference, especially when specialist rehabilitation places are as rare as hen's teeth.

REFERENCES

1. Starfield B. 1994. Is primary care essential? *Lancet* 344:1129–33.
2. Pereira Gray. Towards research-based learning outcomes for general practice in medical schools: Inaugural Barbara Starfield Memorial Lecture. http://dx.doi.org/10.3399/bjgpopen17X100569.
3. Fletcher E, Abel GA, Anderson R et al. 2017. Quitting patient care and career break intentions among general practitioners in South West England: Findings of a census survey of general practitioners. *BMJ Open* 7:015853.
4. British social attitudes survey. 2017. Kings Fund Analysis 2.1.2018. https://www.kingsfund.org.uk/publications/public-satisfaction-nhs-social-care-2018.
5. Matheson C. et al. 2016. Resilience of primary healthcare professionals. *Br J Gen Pract*. DDI:10.3399/BJGP16x685261.
6. Care Quality Commission. 2017. The state of care in general practice 2014–2017 CQC, London.
7. Tudor Hart. 2000. Commentary: Three decades of the inverse care law. *BMJ* 320(7226):18–19.
8. Jackson D, Firtko A and Edenborough M. 2007. Personal resilience as a strategy for surviving and thriving in the face of workplace adversity: A literature review. *J Adv Nurs* 60:1–9.
9. Starey N. 2003. *The Challenge for Primary Care*, Radcliffe Press, ISBN 1-85775-569-3.
10. Tom Lehrer. 1965. *That Was the Week That Was*, Pye Records, R6179 Werner von Braun.
11. House of Commons Health Committee. 2016. Primary care: Fourth report of session 2015–16. HC 408. www.parliament.uk/healthcare.

3

The sector's heritage

INTRODUCTION

The well-developed primary care sector in the United Kingdom is not just an accident of history. Stretching back into the time of the crusades this country has a heritage of charitable and religious foundations, voluntary movements and community initiatives to be proud of. Barbara Starfield points out [1] that a well-developed primary care sector – first point of contact, holistic care to a registered undifferentiated population – is often associated with a more efficient and effective healthcare system overall and in the United Kingdom this long heritage of community-organised healthcare provision has been a sure foundation on which to build. To understand why the UK primary care sector has evolved the way it has, and indeed why it is currently taking on an even more central role both as commissioner of healthcare across the whole National Health Service (NHS) and as provider of an ever-increasing proportion of healthcare, we need to consider the context within which the sector has developed, the forces which have moulded its services and its designers – who have such a rich heritage behind them – for us to build on. If we are to understand how the sector may evolve in the future we need to appreciate how it has developed over time, and why it behaves the way it does – why its culture, its focus, its relationships and its prejudices are driving its current behaviour. This chapter explores the development of some of the elements making up the sector so as to provide some historical perspective to later chapters and is predicated on the principle that we have to learn lessons from the past if we are to build a better future. There is a confounding variable to consider: the world in which the primary care sector has to perform now and into the future is very different from the world it has come from. This does not make consideration of the sector's past irrelevant: our individual emotional, psychological and physical health and beliefs, behaviour and problems continue to evolve at a much slower pace than the industrial, social and digital revolutions which have transformed other aspects of modern life. So consideration of how the sector has developed is no less relevant here than is the study of our history in other situations.

Society in the United Kingdom has changed dramatically during the twentieth century. Following the *industrial* revolution and the social turmoil of the nineteenth century, the twentieth century which produced a *social* revolution. The emancipation of women following World War I is only one example of a trend which saw

- The rise of organised labour
- The emancipation of both men and women through universal primary and secondary education
- A major redistribution of wealth
- Political emancipation through universal suffrage for all adults

All leading to a blurring and gradual disappearance of the class boundaries that had underpinned the British class system for hundreds of years.

This social revolution has fundamentally shaken and changed the values and beliefs which underpinned Victorian society and is of course reflected in similar social revolutions in other countries. Even in Victorian times, health services in the United Kingdom were made up of a partnership between private enterprise, the voluntary sector and public provision. The heritage of Victorian hospitals is a testament to both this public provision and the charitable and voluntary sector, which left us with many of our great teaching institutions as well as endowed wards, beds and cots. The Red Cross, St John Ambulance Association and the tradition of a strong community nursing profession reflect this heritage of community healthcare.

Out-of-hospital services at the beginning of the twentieth century were less organised and less developed than services in the hospital sector. Isolated, single-handed medical practitioners, apothecaries, dentists and pharmacists were not universally available to the whole population whose access to healthcare services depended primarily on the individual's ability to pay, where they lived and their class. The Victorian heritage of "the market" meant it was economic forces that determined an individual's access to healthcare and the population's health status rather than any individual's healthcare needs.

The social revolution during the second half of twentieth century has included a revolution in the primary care sector, which has responded to, and been moulded by the forces unleashed by the revolution elsewhere. In society at large the rapid pace of change throughout the twentieth century. Indeed the increasingly rapid pace of change in the last decades of the century has inevitably challenged the ability of health services to respond and evolve appropriately; technology, emancipation, globalisation and capitalism affect the healthcare sector as much as any other sector of the economy. Individual citizens, professional groups and organisations only change when they have to (Napoleon realised this). Rather than rush into change enthusiastically, most have to be coerced or induced to change. Examples such as the adoption of seat belts and the take up of cervical screening and the reduction of smoking show what can be achieved for the population by systematic, coordinated action over time. The reduction in smoking is the most recent example at the population level: halved from over thirty percent in the 1970s to about seventeen percent now. Such has been the experience of the revolution in out-of-hospital service. But just as King Canute could not hold back the tides by "royal command", you cannot halt the social revolution by individual or professional dictate. The revolution has some way to go to fully empower individuals to have full control over their lives.

THE DESIGNERS

The employed workforce received state-funded primary medical care services under Lloyd George's National Insurance Act of 1911, but their wives and families had to pay [2]. In his 1918 Cavendish Lecture, Bernard Dawson [3], a physician from the London hospital and a wartime military doctor, described how a comprehensive health service could be coordinated. He was invited to chair a consultative council on the future provision of health services and was the first to propose a hierarchical system of primary care centres linked to district hospitals and regional centres linked to university teaching hospitals. Although largely a professionally dominated model based purely on a medical "disease management" view of healthcare provision, this early design left us with two important elements which are still discernible in the British primary care system today [4]:

1. First, the idea of registration and a lifelong medical record resulted from the Lloyd George reforms, and indeed many general practices still retain these traditional Lloyd George envelopes, which, at least in theory, contain the lifelong medical record of every registered patient. In reality these envelopes are largely retained to use for preparing insurance reports in a world where health records are almost completely computerised and stored digitally "online".
2. Second, Dawson recognised that treatment services on their own would be insufficient to ensure the health of the population. The need for health promotion and disease prevention services was highlighted and has become an important part of modern primary care provision. The importance of immunisation to control infectious diseases and of promoting good health to counteract the harmful effects of smoking, alcohol abuse and drug abuse were recognised.

In addition to Lloyd George's National Insurance Act and the medical leadership supplied by Lord Dawson, the interwar years saw some experimentation into the development of primary healthcare teams, such as those linked to urban regeneration schemes in Aberdeen and south London. Increasingly close links between medical practice and nursing in the community were developing through local nursing associations. Their links with hospital nursing, local authority services such as health visiting and general practice were developing.

Although commitment to their profession and "vocation" were important parts of the ethos of all healthcare professions practising in the community, there were important differences in organisation, employment and social status which determined aspect of relationships. Indeed, some of the present-day difficulties in establishing and promoting team working and *integrated care systems* are the result of this history. In the 1920s and 1930s, general practice had to make a profit if doctors were to have an income. Some profit came from registration as a result of the National Insurance Act, while other patients paid for care themselves. General practice was mainly a family business carried out from the doctor's home with little equipment, poor status within the medical profession and little relief from the burden of twenty-four hour, seven days a week duty. This was a *private sector*, small business. Modern-day general practice partners remain self-employed, small business people whose income depends on the profitability of the business they own a share of. *Community nursing* developed alongside but usually in isolation from general practice, although it frequently shared values and commitment to the care of local individuals and communities. In a time when the social order determined a relatively fixed, hierarchical attitude to social status:

- *Doctor's status* – On a pedestal, respected, car-owning, educated and able to sit down with the vicar and the squire.
- *Nurse's status* – Employed by the council or local district nursing association, housed and supported by community funds, uniformed and independent professionals. They lost their housing and pension if they married. They were trained and respected by their patients, but marginalised from the mainstream of the nursing profession which remained hospital based. (See Chapter 1, Box 1.1.)

Similarly, other healthcare practitioners working in the community between the wars – pharmacists, midwives, health visitors, opticians, dentists, dieticians, physiotherapists and occupational therapists, and so on – reflect their heritage and each has developed in relative isolation from each other. For general practice and other contractors such as pharmacists, dentists and opticians, their life and values reflected the private sector – small businesses rooted in the community.

THE BIRTH OF THE NATIONAL HEALTH SERVICE

The 1942 Beveridge Report [5] proposed state funding for the nationalised health service and aimed for universal coverage to tackle the five giants [6] on the road to reconstruction after World War II:

- Want
- Disease
- Ignorance
- Squalor
- Idleness

This report, along with the report of the British Medical Association's (BMA's) Medical Planning Commission in 1942, which also called for a comprehensive service covering the population, made it possible for the post-war labour government to introduce the National Health Service Act in 1946 [7,8]. The service was born into the post-war climate of austerity and shortages made worse by the harsh winter of 1947. The social revolution which had emancipated women and transformed the workforce, housing and education now saw the provision of a National Health Service as an important social priority, alongside nationalisation of core industries, social security, education and housing reforms. Unlike other industrialised Western countries, whose experience of the social revolution in the twentieth century was different, the British "socialist" approach served to marry the differing histories of the professions involved and the institutions and organisations that had previously provided healthcare.

As far as primary care services were concerned, they were seen as peripheral to the main thrust of the NHS Act, which served to develop and nationalise hospital and specialist services. GPs remained self-employed, independent contractors, but provided comprehensive general medical services to the whole population; nurses, midwives and health visitors became state employees; and pharmacists, opticians and dentists worked under similar contractual, national arrangements as general medical practitioners. Primary care services were funded partly from local authority funds and partly from general medical services allocations from Parliament. The original act emphasised the development of health centres [7] which would be built, equipped and staffed at public expense and provide medical, dental and health promotion services plus associated specialist outpatient sessions. Unfortunately, lack of finances meant such centres were rarely provided. The 18,000 GPs, mostly male and over half of them working as single-handed GPs, usually practised from there own homes. Administrative and support staff were mostly entirely lacking (apart from the doctor's wife) and facilities were often rudimentary. The act introduced a Medical Practices Committee, which helped to redistribute GPs, over time, to areas of the country with doctor shortages and to restrict access to areas with excess doctors. It is notable that services in London were frequently of poor quality – costs of provision were higher than elsewhere and specialist hospital services dominated the landscape [9]. I find it remarkable that this pattern of poor quality in London has also been found in the Care Quality Commission's recent inspection programme [10]. Despite the best efforts of everyone involved the quality of general practice in London still lags behind the rest of the country.

A patients guide produced by the Ministry of Health in 1948 [8] said that as everyone could now have a GP, it was that GP who would "arrange for the patient, every kind of specialist care he himself is unable to give. Except in emergencies, hospitals and specialists would not normally accept a patient for advice and treatment unless they had been sent by the family doctor" [8]. This ethos served to institutionalise the referral system and the GP's role as "gatekeeper", which before the NHS had been an arrangement doctors aimed for. With the establishment of the NHS, gatekeeping served as an effective way of controlling patient demand and ensuring the protection of specialist services. This gatekeeping system reinforced the separation of primary and secondary care with the referral letter and the discharge summary being the currency of transfer between the sectors. Family doctors defended the system because through it they had continuing responsibility for the individual patient, consultants defended it because it protected them from cases they might consider trivial or outside their field of interest, and the government defended it because it saved money to have a filter in the system. The fundamental relationship between GP and specialist had been altered. Previously, specialists made most of their money from private practice and therefore courted GPs for referrals; after the establishment of the NHS, specialists had less need to court GPs for private work but also had little reason to be grateful to them for deluging them with NHS referrals.

THE DYNAMICS

The birth of the NHS into the austere, resource-constrained, battered and bruised post-war British society cannot be considered as an isolated event. Rather, the birth followed a long gestation:

- From the long history of healthcare and welfare support in the country – from the hospitallers time of the Crusades through the services provided by religious orders and monasteries through to the time of the Industrial Revolution and the need to ensure the fitness of the workforce and the armed services through a more organised approach to medical and nursing care provision.
- From the forces released by the social revolution, which liberated British people from
  - The suppression of personal conscientiousness resulting from lifelong servitude.
  - The exclusion of half the population from full participation in the affairs of the country until women's emancipation after World War I.
  - The distortions of the class system which affected access to education, health services and economic resources as well as power.
    - The crisis of identity which crumbling British imperialism faced as a result of two World Wars and their effect on the values and vigour of the nation.

The founding principles of the welfare state, outlined in the Beveridge Report [5], specified that the nation had a responsibility to the population *as a community* – a responsibility to invest during the good times to ensure that the weak, the sick, the elderly and the socially disadvantaged would be looked after in their time of need, implying an end to the exaggerations of market forces having free reign over welfare issues. While important in themselves, developments such as the NHS Act, the Dawson Report [3] and the Beveridge Report [5] were merely stages in the process of individual liberation, communal social responsibility, which the social revolution of the twentieth century released.

Of course, such energies can either be directed constructively or can conflict with each other to inhibit progress. In physiological processes, the individual elements of a system are linked together and are dependent on each other for success. Similar principles apply in industrial systems, education, and so on. All of these systems require energy to drive them and are controlled by feedback arrangements so that the efficiency and effectiveness of the system are maximised.

In these terms, the birth of the NHS can be considered as the logical response or intervention by the British community to the forces released by the social revolution and the necessity to revalue the resources of the nation following the predations of war. The NHS was therefore a service developed as a response to a dynamic system or situation and was designed to be

- Responsive to community requirements
- Sensitive to technological change and evolving social requirements
- Constantly changing and evolving in response to circumstances

However, the dynamic system that the NHS was designed to drive has failed to respond to these forces appropriately:

- The community requirements have changed. A world at peace is focussing on international relationships, global warming, migration and populism, and the NHS – popular though it is with the population – is no longer being driven by national policy. Rather the NHS has become like a national religion – impossible for politicians to constrain and redirect, and like a cuckoo in the nest consuming more and more of the nation's resources at the expense of other competing priorities.
- Technological and social changes of the last seventy years have transformed the context within which healthcare is delivered opened new treatment possibilities and new models of accessing and providing care.
- The NHS has become stuck in an inflexible design which is no longer responsive to circumstances. Basically, the original NHS Mk 1 is no longer fit for its purpose, but managers, clinicians and politicians have proven unable to lead the service. Constant tinkering with structures without reforming processes has not been effective or sufficiently radical.

PRIMARY CARE: 1950–2000

The NHS Act (1946) [7] translated the work of the earlier "designers" of health services into a truly national service. For the first time, the NHS gave the whole population the right of access, free at the point of use, to a general practitioner or family doctor. The unique position of the family doctor as the patient's advocate and as gatekeeper to the rest of the health and welfare service was designed in from the start. The doctor's role was to act both as an independent counterweight to a centralised, bureaucratic and impersonal service, and as a care coordinator, controlling or regulating access to specialist services.

Universal registration through a national contract with highly centralised administration was the process by which the national service was established, along with the associated redistribution of resources and clear definition of the patient's and practitioner's rights and responsibilities. A continuation of the registration cards originally introduced by Lloyd George (and in the author's experience still treasured by those who were entitled to them in the years between the two World Wars) helped to symbolise the universal enfranchisement that the NHS introduced. General practice and in particular general medical practitioners, by virtue of registration and gatekeeping, became the most powerful players in the primary care sector at the birth of the NHS. *Although we need to reflect that if power is the ability to do things, then at the birth of the NHS these powers were quite limited. Compared to the present day, the general practitioner had a limited formulary to prescribe from, limited diagnostic equipment, no ancillary staff and no nursing or other qualified practitioner support.* Inevitably, in the sea of pathology that the NHS inherited, disease management rather than health promotion or the prevention of disease was the top priority and, therefore, the pre-eminence of the "medical model" was entirely understandable. The pre-eminence of the medical model did, however, mean that primary and community nursing, dentistry, ophthalmic services and the professions allied to medicine were only empowered "second hand" and became dependent on the medical model for their influence. Patients were essentially "supplicant" – more dependent on the doctor's ethical behaviour than before the NHS, as they were no longer paying directly for the service.

An early report into the state of general practice was funded by the Nuffield Trust in 1948. Dr Joseph Collins surveyed a variety of English practices and found great variation in their standards [9]. In city practices he saw no examples of effective practice and described surgeries without any facilities for examining patients, without any systematic record-keeping and without any facilities for proper consultation. The country doctor tended to know his patients better and to spend more time with them. Many GPs seemed to be competent and effective clinicians, but, taken as a whole, the report was a damning indictment of the state of English general practice. There seemed to be no definition of quality of care and no standards against which to monitor performance. Collins noted that the worst practices tended to be found where the populations need was greatest and that good quality practices tended to be in areas farthest away from large hospitals. Some premises required condemnation in the public interest. Collins recommended the establishment of primary care teams, linking doctors, nurses, social workers and technicians in group practices serving 15,000–20,000 people. He blamed the widening gap between hospital and primary care on the lack of political interest at local and national levels, and on the failure of the national GP contract and nationalised administration to invest in the development of primary care services [9].

The Collins article was followed by the BMA-sponsored Hadfield survey [11] and the Taylor survey [12] on good general practice: "In the final analysis, quality of the service depends on the men and women who are actually doing the job". The response to these early reports pointing out the weakness of the primary care sector was to increase investment such as recommended by Danckwerts' proposals [13], which moved remuneration away from a flat capitation rate and introduced a basic practice allowance and financial encouragement for single-handed practitioners to form partnerships and group practices. A more even distribution of doctors was being encouraged by the Medical Practices Committee and there was a steady decrease in the number of patients living in areas of doctor shortage through the early 1950s. The Royal College of General Practitioners (RCGP) was established so that family medicine with its own skills and knowledge base, would have its own academic body, curriculum, research and college to promote it. As early as 1952, Health Minister Iain McCloud [13] called for investment in general practice in order to improve its status, be of benefit to patients and cut waiting lists. He encouraged the development of group practices and primary care teams, including midwives, district nurses and health visitors, and closer working with dentists, pharmacists and opticians. Thus the vision from the minister, the nascent RCGP and further government investment began the renaissance of general practice in the mid to late 1950s.

Taken together this history represents an analysis of general practice as a part of the primary care system in the early years of the NHS and how leverage from systematic enquiry, publication and lobbying, developed a framework of incentives through which the sector could develop – leverage could be applied to change the system.

Towards the end of the 1950s and throughout the 1960s, the development of training courses for GPs received more attention. The College of General Practitioners [14], coordinated by John Horder, recommended two years postgraduate education in supervised general practice and three years in hospital posts. Horder also recommended the establishment of academic departments of general practice in every medical school. These were moves to establish the discipline of general practice, but were restricted to general medical practice rather than including the other disciplines involved in the primary care sector – nursing, dentistry, pharmacy, and so on. This meant that the development of professional practice in these other disciplines received less consideration and investment. Naturally the development of new drugs and the expansion of the pharmaceutical industry meant that community pharmacy and its relationship with the NHS became more important. Advertising and pharmaceutical representatives focussed on general practitioners as "prescribers", and sponsorship of postgraduate education by the industry also bought influence. This was the era of rapid expansion in the availability of new effective medicines – antibiotics, benzodiazepines, beta-blockers, and so on – which began to transform the range of medication available to the population so that their health problems could be managed within primary care.

So the range of healthcare that could be offered to people by the primary care sector expanded, but not by general practice in isolation. The sector was dependent on cooperation between all the clinical disciplines for its provision of holistic care.

The system through which general practices were paid did little to reward high-quality practice and by the early 1960s an additional review considering the future of family practice was required. The essential feature of the pool system was that almost all payment was made from a national pool without any consideration of

- The health needs of local communities
- The range of services offered by the practice
- The costs of providing those services

There was therefore little encouragement for practices to invest in developing better services for patients and little reward for providing better care. And because the income of the self-employed, independent contractor, GPs remained entirely dependent on the profits of their practices. There was little incentive for them to invest in the business if it did not increase the profits.

Leverage – or an incentive framework – was needed to improve the quality of care patients received by encouraging GPs to invest in developing their practices.

A further review, *The Field of Work of the Family Doctor* [15], looked ahead to what the family doctor was likely to be doing over the succeeding ten to fifteen years and served to lay the foundations for the development of the primary care sector. In it the author Gillie saw the GP of the future as the coordinator of the application of the resources between hospital and community care, that is, the effective gatekeeper. Although not universally welcomed by all GPs, the Gillie Report formed the backdrop to negotiations with the Wilson (labour) government in 1964 when Kenneth Robinson, as Minister of Health, negotiated the 1966 GPs charter with Dr James Cameron (the BMA General Medical Services Committee chairman). This charter, negotiated in difficult national economic circumstances, turned the tide in general practice. The number of GPs recruited began to rise, investment in premises and in the development of primary care teams expanded, and incentives to improve the quality of care patients received were welcomed. There was an upsurge of interest in health centres, the development of GP training and postgraduate education centres – usually based in hospitals.

Although sometimes described as a seminal event, the 1966 charter is better described as another turn of the evolutionary wheel – a step towards the dynamic, high-quality, responsive system the community requires and an adaptation to support the primary care sector in providing the expanded range of services that technological advances permitted. However this charter was evolutionary in its approach – like introducing a "better Morris Minor" rather than transformative – leaping to new design featuring new primary care organisations, new relationships, flexible local contracting arrangements and systematic career support for practitioners.

In 1962, the report of the BMA's 1958 Committee of Enquiry into the NHS, chaired by Sir Arthur Porritt [16], was published. It supported the continued development of the NHS as a state-funded monopoly, encouraging private practice in order to challenge the state monopoly's tendency to sloth and indolence and to protect professional freedom. The report supported the continuation of the tripartite funding arrangements (see earlier) but suggested that the services should be brought together under a single Area Board so that management across local authority, hospital and primary care could be better coordinated. This report, alongside the Gillie Report, prepared the ground for the development of the NHS for the next ten to fifteen years. The agreement between the GPs and the government, leading to the new GP contract in 1966, secured new funding for primary care teams, supporting professional practice and improved services for patients. The move from single-handed practice to partnerships with the employment of administrative and secretarial support and practice nurses was promoted along with the development of purpose-built premises, continuing professional development and some incentives to provide a broader range of services to a smaller population through "item of service fees" forming a larger proportion of income. Unfortunately, as with all negotiated solutions, there were some compromises in the charter. The financial arrangements, the "pool", did not radically shift resources to tackle health problems and health inequalities or to reward high-quality innovative practice. In addition, the charter focussed on general practice but was not matched by similar arrangements for other independent contractors, district nurses, health visitors or midwives. The charter did not look at the role of general practitioners working in hospitals and did not consider the coordination of primary care, hospital care and local authority services in a way that addressed the needs of individuals in the community for coordinated healthcare. The role of general practice in promoting the health of the community (the public health role) similarly remained under developed. General practice, the primary care team and the broader primary care workforce continued to focus on the management of disease, remaining reactive to the demands of individual patients and relatively isolated for the rest of the NHS. The administration of general practice and other independent contractors remained the responsibility of the "Executive Committee" and was not integrated with the management of the rest of the NHS as recommended by the Porritt Committee.

Because the development of the system has been "stepped" rather than continuous – intervention, report, intervention, and so on – it has always been subject to interruption and manipulation as a result of economic or political pressures.

For many GPs, the years following the 1966 charter were regarded as a golden age of new investment, administrative support, better premises and better support for professional practice with training programmes and continuous professional development. Nevertheless workloads remained heavy and the relative professional isolation of practitioners meant variations in the standard of care people received. In addition, the active questioning of the power of the medical profession and the paternalistic relationship between doctor and patient had begun. Illich [17] articulated and interpreted the risks involved to all sides, while access to television programmes fuelled public understanding of health issues and demystified medicine. The economic constraints of the 1970s, with inflation, fuel supply crises and industrial unrest, affected the NHS as much as any other sector of society, so that while the 1966 charter introduced much needed investment and reform, general practice and the broader primary care sector were not liberated to grow and develop in isolation from the broader developments in society. In addition technological change introduced new therapies enabling treatment at home, for example treatment of peptic ulcers and home dialysis and shorter length of stay in hospital. The process of de-institutionalisation began and has gone on to affect care of the elderly, mental health and learning disability care, as well as care in acute hospitals. These processes have changed the nature of primary healthcare and challenged many of the professional roles and responsibilities involved in the sector. But the sector's design still reflected its small shopkeeper, medical model approach – the Morris Minor lived on, even if now fitted with seat belts and disk brakes.

So technological and social changes and the forces they release also affect development – increasing life expectancy, smaller families and urbanisation all play their part.

The late 1970s and early 1980s saw further reviews of general practice, with attempts to tackle variation in quality and the emerging need to develop health promotion and disease prevention within primary care, as well as providing effective management of acute and chronic disease. Sadly, political posturing and the intransigence of GP negotiators inhibited progress. The lack of effective leadership to address "quality" and "improving health" agendas meant that little progress was made in providing a more effective primary care sector to meet the needs of the population during the 1980s. The internal market, a new GP contract in 1990 and the introduction of GP fundholding brought some new dynamism into the primary care sector, challenging traditional planning models and introducing more focus on local circumstances and market forces. Unfortunately, the issues of fairness and responsiveness to the varying needs of individuals and populations were not adequately dealt with. The internal market and GP fundholding challenged many practitioners' views of social responsibility and the purpose of the health service, and, in pure economic terms, the jury remained undecided about the benefits of the reforms until they were swept away by the election of the labour government in 1997 [18]. Nevertheless, the legacy of the conservative reforms of the 1990s in preparing the primary care sector for the challenges of the modern world should not be ignored:

- The moves towards corpocracy
- The understanding of the need for different more open and accountable governing arrangements
- The need for team working and planning in the primary care sector
- The changing relationship between consumers of healthcare and the professions providing that care

It would not be right to end this consideration of the heritage of the primary care sector without considering some of the gaps which remained when the Labour government came to power in 1997 and which have left a legacy behind them.

MANAGEMENT OF THE PRIMARY CARE SECTOR

As described earlier, the primary care sector from the start of the NHS has been built around a business model characterised by

- Independent small businesses, usually run by professional partnerships, largely self-capitalising but reliant on the NHS for income.
- Informal working arrangements with other care providers in the community, relying on personal relationships rather than formal contracts or agreements to arrange and agree on working practices.
- The absence of any planned approach to service development beyond nationally agreed contracting arrangements. No coordinated sectorwide and intersector mechanisms for agreeing and delivering service improvements.
- Autonomous – not open to scrutiny or accountable for resource utilisation or performance. No publication of performance data, no scrutiny of results or performance, and no effective governance framework for ensuring the trustworthiness of clinical or organisational performance.

Until 1984, independent contractor provider organisations – GP practices, opticians, dentists and pharmacists –were administered by the local executive committees which dealt with registration, contractor payments and the administration of the national contracts. Their successor bodies – the Family Practitioner Committee (FPC) from 1984 to 1990 and the Family Health Service Authority (FHSA) from 1990 to 1995 – continued to administer rather than manage the sector.

Roy Griffiths's [19] inquiry into NHS management had recommended the introduction of general management into the NHS in 1983, but did not consider management in the primary care sector. General management was rapidly introduced at national, regional, district and hospital (unit) levels. The impact of general management in terms of leadership, accountability and professional management practice has been great, and the associated development of clinical leadership through clinical directorships has helped to ensure that management priorities are tempered by clinical insight. But the absence of the primary care sector from this axis of power has been unfortunate. The consequent lack of management focus on the sector for the intervening thirty-five years has meant

- A lack of understanding of the way the primary care sector works or of the values and cultural norms which govern performance in the sector.
- A lack of investment in capacity and infrastructure – a problem when the "scope of practice" has been rapidly expanding.
- A lack of leadership development programmes for both managers and clinicians meaning that confidence in the ability of the sector to deliver on its responsibilities has been lacking throughout NHS.
- A lack of support for organisational development both in small businesses and at locality levels including issues of governance and cohesion.

When the health authorities introduced in 1995 took over responsibility for the primary care sector from FHSAs, they did so without adequate experience and understanding of the culture of the primary care sector, and many continued to focus their attention on the hospital sector and the imperatives of the annual local contracting round. The task of developing a primary care sector equipped for its future responsibilities, tackling the variation in quality in the sector, ensuring safe care and holding providers to account for their performance was left largely "on one side".

Primary care trusts (PCTs) inherited responsibilities from health authorities in 2001 and continued to be responsible for the local administration and management of the NHS until 2013 when clinical commissioning groups (CCGs) took over. Most local hospitals had become self-governing "Foundation Trusts" in the early years of PCTs and when the "provider" arms of PCTs (community nursing and associated services) were incorporated into "community NHS trusts", PCTs were able to begin the process of transforming the primary care sector and introducing a planned care approach to support best clinical practice. While PCTs and CCGs have had responsibility for commissioning care through NHS trusts, they still only have responsibility for administering the nationally negotiated contracts in the primary care sector.

The national contracting framework for general medical practice has continued to support the small shopkeeper business model, but with some variation through alternative provider medical services (APMS) and personal medical services (PMS) variants, and the BMA's GP Committee successfully agreed with NHS England and implemented developments such as the following:

- The 2004 new GMS contract
  - Introduced a "Quality and Outcomes Framework" (QOF) to incentivise systematic care for some people with long-term conditions such as asthma, hypertension and diabetes.
  - Effectively relieved GPs of responsibility for providing "out-of-hours" care, which is now provided through providers commissioned through CCGs – either derivatives of previous GP cooperative arrangements or private sector providers.
- Expanded access arrangements to open new opportunities for patients – walk-in centres and private GP surgeries in railway stations for example.
- The introduction of telephone triage arrangements – initially NHS direct and more recently NHS 111.

However, the decade of national economic austerity has significantly affected development of the sector. Despite the development of the NHSE's *Five Year Forward View* [21] and the associated *GP Forward View* [22], with their promise of new investment, most resources have continued to be diverted to bolster the balance sheets of hospital trusts.

Centrally developed and monitored programmes such as "Vanguard" projects to test "new models of care" (NMC); sustainability and transformation plans (STPs); and accountable care systems (ACSs), accountable care organisations (ACOs) and integrated care systems (ICSs) all represent attempts by the NHS to adapt to the requirements of austerity by improving the efficiency and effectiveness of care provision, but in an environment where general practice and the whole primary care sector is struggling to cope with the demands placed on them. To the extent that the resilience and sustainability of general practice and the primary care sector is threatened, we have to be concerned that these moves to learn about NMC and ACOs/ICSs are not addressing the full agenda.

The consequences of the years of austerity, the decades of marginalisation and the heritage of independent practice include:

- Difficulty in recruiting and retaining the required workforce. The *Five Year Forward View* promised 5000 more GPs, but 2017 saw a net loss of 700 GP partners in England.
- The greatest percentage fall in the confidence that users have in General Practice in the thirty-five years of the British Social Attitudes survey [23] by seven percent between 2016 and 2017 to sixty-five percent.
- Falling profitability in the sector. Data is not collected centrally, but unpublished local data suggests that GP partners "take-home" pay, the only section of the GP workforce which is affected by falling profitability, may have fallen by over twenty percent in the last decade at a time when the rest of the workforce has also been constrained to less than inflation increases in income.
- An increasing workload. The King's Fund quarterly monitoring report June 2017 [24] reported a 7.5% rise in consultation rates over the previous 2 years in its survey of 200 practices. This increasing workload is driven by the ageing population and restricted access to care elsewhere in the health service.

This is not a picture to inspire confidence in the future. The House of Commons Select Committee Enquiry into the sector [25] made useful recommendations about capacity, access and workforce planning. But without a coherent vision for the future of the sector or one that is recognised by the sector's stakeholders as inspiring sufficient confidence in the future to restore public trust and workforce motivation, the sector is left feeling underdressed for the party.

Before ending our look at the heritage the sector inherited from its designers, we need to also consider how fit other consequences of its heritage are for the future.

MANAGEMENT OF GP PRACTICES

1. *The role of the partnership*: The organisational form of most UK general practices is that of a professional partnership – similar to other community professions such as solicitors and accountants. As general practitioners started to move away from single-handed practice through the 1950s and 1960s they formed into organisations which employed staff, developed premises, agreed on joint working arrangements, and their scope and approach to practice. As "directors" of the business, the partners lived by dividing the "profits" the business made among the directors in the proportion of the share they each hold in the business and make the decisions and are responsible to each other for delivering the business. This remains the dominant organisational form in the sector, but it has struggled to adapt to the following:

   * The kind of approach to corporate governance that has influenced other parts of the public sector and private business [20], which seeks to promote trust between the business and its users by introducing arrangements that ensure openness and accountability, balance executive power with non-executive challenges, and separate the role of the chair from that of the chief executive. Whereas in small partnerships some aspects might be seen as unnecessary, as practices have grown so the trust and confidence that they enjoy needs to be reinforced.
   * Because the partners share the profits generated by the business in proportions – or shares – they agree that they may not all be "equal" partners and this may cause some imbalance in power within the business.
   * The partnership is not time limited. There is no annual or three-yearly cycle, partners leave when they retire from the business, or when the business account is settled. This makes it quite an inflexible arrangement for adapting to changing circumstances, such as family or career development.
   * Partners are interdependent; they have to trust each other. When finance or performance is "stressed", tensions within partnerships can be inflamed. In the past this frequently led to partnership splits and years of acrimonious relationships to the detriment of sector harmony.
   * As partnerships are inherently inward looking, they have struggled to respond to the changing needs of the rest of the NHS and the community they exist within. It has only been when the forces bringing them together

have exceeded the forces keeping them separate, such as around sharing care for each other's patients outside normal "office" hours and benefits of joint working are realised. Federating or merging into larger partnerships or moving into arrangements with corporate bodies to "support" practice development have all become attractive options for partnerships, particularly for those facing challenging circumstances.

* The history of general practice has been largely within the practice of medicine, with employed nurses and loose joint working with other clinicians in the community, but decision-making power has been largely owned by the GP partners. Arrangements to support nurses, practice managers or pharmacists to become active shareholding partners in the business have been tried, but they remain very unusual. Because of the dominance of the GP partners there has been an imbalance of power within the system, resentment by "employed" staff – be they "salaried" doctors, practice nurses, pharmacists or practice managers – about being excluded from when decisions are made is sometimes vocalised but more commonly felt.

* The voice of the community, be that NHS commissioners or users of the service, patients or their representatives is only heard indirectly. They have no voice, only influence. This lack of "user empowerment" – to mirror what has happened elsewhere in the public sector, like parent governors in schools, non-executive members of NHS boards and elected local authority councillors – have wrongly fossilised the relationship between service provider and user in the pattern of NHS in the 1950s rather than reflecting the realities of modern society.

2. *The role of the practice manager*: During the 1970s and 1980s more practices found themselves struggling to administer their business – the complexities of the national GMS contract – detailed in the "red book". The problems of employing staff and maintaining premises, keeping records, and managing complaints and appointment systems, all tasks that had to be fitted around surgeries and home visits and tasks partners had not been trained to undertake and sometimes struggled to do successfully. The development of a practice manager was a response to these pressures. Sometimes there was an external appointment of someone with general management skills from another sector, but commonly it was an internal appointment of a member of staff with knowledge of the practice, but often not of the external environment.

Over recent years the role of the practice manager has become more established. Training courses and support networks, close working with other organisations such as NHS bodies, and local community groups have joined with their other general management responsibilities to make them a central player in the success of the practice. But:

* They have usually remained as employees of the business rather than partners or directors, so while many will attend partners meetings they struggle to ensure that partners recognise the importance of their roles and responsibilities and the different but complementary roles of managers and partners.

- They have limited support from the rest of the NHS. Performance review and appraisal is usually managed within the practice, further training and development is a practice prerogative, and career development opportunities are limited.

3. *Corporate and social enterprise management of GP practice*: In recent years, some practices have sought outside help to support them in meeting the challenges they face. Sometimes this help was from companies started by entrepreneurial GPs, sometimes by businesses from other sectors looking for a business opportunity and sometimes as social enterprise initiatives from within the local community. These new providers either worked alongside the partnership through an existing GMS contract or more commonly an APMS arrangement with the NHS to meet particular local needs, such as when a partnership failed or when a particular local need required a new practice to be formed for meeting the needs of the homeless or refugees, for example.

Some of these arrangements have been successful and been rated as "outstanding" by the Care Quality Commission, but too many have struggled.

- They have taken over "damaged goods", that is, practices with a history of poor performance, poor reputation and low morale, and the new provider, often with the best of intentions, has found that cultural change is very difficult. Too often retained staff and existing patients remain stuck in historic poor-performance cycles. Even considerable investment may only produce temporary cosmetic change.
- Providers with a distant headquarters servicing the needs of a range of healthcare providers often develop a corporate portfolio of policies and systems through which they implement their service model. While this can helpfully introduce a more systematic and standardised management platform it has been found to be less successful in reinforcing trust between the practice and its stakeholders and less successful in improving the quality of clinical care provided and the measures of clinical efficiency and effectiveness.
- Similarly, corporate providers of out-of-hours care, of minor injury units and walk-in centres, and of online services have faced difficulties over clinical and corporate governance, ensuring safe care and providing high-quality leadership.

Issues for doctors in primary care

1. To develop and share a vision of what being a GP or family doctor means in the modern digital world which can become a narrative to inspire doctors to commit their career to the work and can restore pride to current GPs so that salaried and locum GPs decide to join the permanent workforce.
2. To redefine the "scope of practice" of the GP, family doctor or primary care physician to reflect the multidisciplinary primary care team's expertise and experience, and which recognises the unique contribution the doctor can make

to diagnosing the illness or illnesses the individual is suffering from; making or supporting decision making to detail an appropriate plan of care for the individual; providing biographical care over time for each registered individual so that an ongoing relationship can be built on the basis of trust; managing, on behalf of the individual, the complex care pathway that is involved in helping the individual cope with multi-morbidity, frailty and vulnerability.

3. To recognise that this scope of practice has to be rebalanced to address the inverse care law [26], the public health priorities of the nation (smoking, cancer, obesity, diabetes, dementia, drug addiction and alcohol), and the forgotten long-term conditions, and those excluded from systematic care though the quality and outcomes framework, such as those with sensory diseases such as visual impairment or deafness, those with congenital abnormalities, those with multiple sclerosis or motor neurone disease, those with psoriasis and eczema … this list could go on.

4. Clarify the boundaries between the "expert generalist" and the "specialist" where they work so that shared care of individuals is promoted across professional and organisational boundaries.

5. Adapt to the modern world by ensuring that the benefits of digital technology; a shared, common healthcare record; self-care by empowered individual patients; and remote clinical monitoring are promoted, but in an evidence-based, safe and efficient fashion to minimise risk.

6. To free themselves from the shackles of historic protectionist practice and grasp the opportunities to lead the development of health and welfare services unconstrained by the myopia of dinosaurs.

7. To recognise that poor performance, be it individual or organisational inadequacy, is a risk for all GPs. It can only be avoided if isolationist tendencies are avoided and professionalism is constantly revalued, either by a systematic approach to regular clinical supervision or by a systematic programme of professional inspection.

8. To insist that best practice in the rest of the NHS is essential in the primary care sector, for example including infection control, health and safety, career development, appraisal, human resource management, and all aspects of clinical and corporate governance.

9. To build links with the communities they serve so that the role of the doctor as teacher is re-established to empower individuals to learn about their own health and take responsibility for managing the issues they face.

10. To ensure that their scope of practice drives a scheme of delegation towards "Doctors do what only doctors can do" and "Nurses do what only nurses can do". Where the needs of individuals and their families
    * Are met by who is most qualified to meet them. The GP should no longer be the only go-to person.
    * Are held together by the "golden thread" of an integrated, biographical, lifelong healthcare record available to all contacts between the individual and their clinicians and carers.
    * Provide the context for decision making about clinical care whenever and wherever required – individual needs are at the centre of the system.

NURSING

The three branches of the nursing profession working in the community – district nursing, midwifery and health visiting – have long and honourable histories. While district nursing often remained the responsibility of the voluntary sector, with local district nursing associations funding the local service, health visiting has a history based in radical local politics and the development of community services by local authorities. The public health function of health visitors, that is, preventing disease and promoting health through improved sanitation and personal behaviour, has long been part of the health visiting philosophy. Midwifery is really a separate profession from nursing, although many nurses take it up. Between the wars, the great majority of births took place at home supervised by midwives who would call for medical support only if complications developed. Although in rural areas nurses might be "triple qualified", fulfilling midwifery, health visiting and district nursing duties, in most places the three services operated separately and not always harmoniously. The working conditions of each service were determined by their employers and could be quite different. District nurses, for example, were often not permitted to marry, and if they did they risked losing their home, their job and their pension. Health visitors, employed by local authorities, were treated very differently.

Nursing in the community has developed informally as an extension of family care since the original "poor laws" in the time of Elizabeth I. More formally, outreach of religious orders during the early nineteenth century and then the establishment of the district nursing service in the 1850s reflected the changes in society of the time. The need for a healthier workforce, the Victorian virtue of charitable giving and voluntary effort, and the emerging relationship between free enterprise and individual responsibility were influential.

Just as pharmacy established itself as a profession separate from medicine during the nineteenth century's Industrial Revolution, with a separate educational, regulatory, ethical and organisational basis, so too did nursing.

From their early beginnings in the 1850s, both district nursing and health visiting followed an employed model rather than a self-employed or "small shopkeeper" model. Employment was with local authorities or voluntary nursing associations, and management was either with the medical officer of health or through senior nurses in the county nursing associations. The traditional role of the district nurse is the provision of "personal care". Illness creates dependency: the sick need not only medical treatment involving diagnosis, therapy and monitoring until recovery but also personal care. The provision of these services and the administration of treatment that the doctor prescribes have been the two basic duties of the nurse. By their skilful care the sick can be restored to health [27].

Health visiting represents an extension to this role, as it has evolved to support the healthy rather than treat the sick. Fulfilling an executive public health function, health visitors from the 1850s have had an educational and advisory function in support of social change. Promoting healthy behaviour and tackling poor sanitation has meant that their knowledge base and training is more about counselling and teaching than about practical nursing. Nevertheless, their effectiveness at tackling infant mortality, breastfeeding, immunisation and child protection is difficult to separate from the efforts of others and of wider social change.

Other branches of the nursing profession have also evolved in response to the industrial and social revolutions. School nursing was first introduced during the Boer War, as it was recognised that the health status of school children left much to be desired. Community psychiatric nursing has evolved largely as an outreach service from specialist mental health provision as a response to the changing pattern of care for people with mental health problems – particularly as long-stay institutional care has transferred to "care in the community". Care of the dying at home has also developed rapidly in recent years as the specialist hospice movement has recognised the need to support people with terminal illness and their families at home.

The establishment of a nursing register (1923) by the Royal College of Nursing of formal education encompassing both theory and practice, and the development of an appropriate career structure reflecting specialist interests and responsibilities have largely developed during the time of the NHS.

The emergence of nurses employed by general practitioners during the 1970s (practice nurses) added another dimension to nursing in primary care. These "treatment room" nurses helped move general practice from its traditional disease management focus towards a more systematic approach to chronic disease management, the prevention of disease and the promotion of better health in the population. Nevertheless the lack of appropriate training programmes, a structure for nurses to advance their career in the sector and membership of the decision-making forums in the practice has meant that practice nursing has attracted nurses whose ambition is more limited than those seeking advancement in a hierarchical, more structured career such as hospital, district nursing or health visiting.

In recent years, practice nursing has developed further through training programmes for nurse practitioners and advanced nurse practitioners, nurse prescribers, and for nurses with special interests, for example in diabetes or respiratory disease. The technical and consulting skills these nurses have brought to the sector are highly valued by patients as well as practices.

These different branches of primary care nursing, along with others such as community midwifery; specialist outreach teams such as for renal dialysis, cancer and neurological disease; alongside voluntary sector nursing services such as the Red Cross, them make up a very heterogeneous primary care nursing profession – with very different cultures, employment status and responsibilities. The concept that they are all nurses is often less strongly adhered to than in the medical profession. Rather, nurses identify more with the branch of the nursing profession to which they belong and give more loyalty to that branch. This fragmentation, which has been perpetuated through the different employment arrangements and different career structures of the branches, is now being challenged by the emergence of a more coherent primary care sector designed to meet the needs of the community for home-based medical and nursing services.

In moving from a national service focussed on disease management to a national system focussing on health, nursing is being transformed from a caring, personal service orientation. Where it is going is less clear – but nurse triage, nurse prescribing and increasing autonomy and power over their scope of practice al help to redefine the professional role of nursing as the primary care sector develops.

Issues for nursing in primary care

(See Chapter 1, Box 1.1 for illustration.)

1. Coordination of nursing provisions across cultural and organisational boundaries so that the nursing care people receive at home is assured, by design.
2. The move beyond an operational provision of care – template and protocol, policy, and practice driven – towards a service which assesses the needs of individuals and works in a team with other healthcare professionals to ensure those needs are met. Through this to add value to care rather than be seen as a cheap alternative to doctor-provided care.
3. To consider the place for nurse leadership of primary care organisations and practice, such as perhaps director of primary care nursing on the board of the provider with responsibility for all nursing provision.
4. To deliver a career pathway for nursing in the sector, from nurse training to specialist practice.
5. To support the delivery of the nation's agenda for improving the health of the community though focussing on key priority areas, such as cancer, smoking, obesity, dementia and addiction.
6. To address the health needs of vulnerable members of the community, that is, the homeless, refugees, the frail elderly and young families.
7. Tackle the areas of identified weakness in healthcare provision in the community, for example, the benefits of breastfeeding have been well known for many years [28] but the proportion of mothers who breastfeed their children has remained too low. At twelve months only 0.5 percent of mothers are still breastfeeding, whereas the figure in Germany is 23 percent, the United States is 27 percent, Brazil is 56 percent and Senegal is 99 percent.

PHARMACY

Background

The separation of pharmacists from doctors started in the eighteenth century when the growing prosperity of the population led to people buy pharmaceutical products and seek advice about their health from chemists and druggists as well as from apothecaries.

The separation of pharmacy from the medical profession with all the associated governing arrangements, for example, registration, control of power, accountability and supervision, developed through the pharmacy acts of the nineteenth century [29] led to the emergence of a strong retail community pharmacy sector in the early twentieth century. The hospital pharmacy developed with the hospital sector but had its roots in the legacy of the poor law hospitals, and was provided either as an add-on to a community pharmacy, or as a stand-alone but rather isolated service until the establishment of the NHS.

Although pharmacists' main business has traditionally been management of medicines, they have throughout the last 200 years also advised patients about their minor ailments and undertaken tasks such as cupping and bleeding, providing surgical supplies, taking weights and blood pressures, and surgical and anaesthetics services. Thus, although the profession has separated culturally from medicine, there remains strong links between them.

The separation of the prescribing of medicines from the dispensing of them started in 1852, but became more important with the Lloyd George National Insurance Act (1911) which served to reinforce the extent to which the pharmacists' incomes were dependent upon the prescribing behaviour of the medical profession.

The growth of the healthcare industry throughout the twentieth century did not leave the pharmacy profession unaffected. The social revolution following the Industrial Revolution, along with the tremendous growth of the multinational pharmaceutical industry, had profound implications. Pharmacists, as graduates, are trained in pharmacology and therapeutics, and understand medicines and how they work. They are not trained to diagnose and manage medical conditions, or in pathology or other aspects of medicine.

The growth in "multiple" stores and supermarket pharmacies has led to the future of the independent, retail, corner shop pharmacy being less secure. The accessibility of such pharmacies seems less of an attraction for the population than the economy of scale offered by supermarkets. The ending of retail price maintenance has further eroded the power base of the independent; the increasing importance of digital pharmacy and the reductions in NHS dispensing fees are now additional factors signalling profound change in the sector. I think we can look forward to a few years to a time when the supply of medicines will be largely from the internet via digital pharmacies which deliver direct to people who request them.

Clinical pharmacy in primary care

As we move through the twenty-first century, pharmacists working in the primary care sector are continuing to adapt to the changing world in which they are carving out their careers. They no longer manufacture drugs, they have had much of their dispensing role automated, and they have remained rather isolated from the development of primary care teams, and latterly from corporate organisations in the primary care sector.

The development of clinical pharmacy services, such as those in hospitals where pharmacists are intimately involved with the provision and supervision of medicines, has been gradually developing in the primary care sector. Pharmaceutical advisers to health authorities have usually been hospital pharmacists with training in clinical pharmacy and are aware of the potential for community pharmacists to develop this role in the primary care sector. The rapid growth in the drug budgets of the NHS (£6.2 billion in 1999/2000) is an important driver towards the development of effective medicines management in the community. The implications for the future of the profession of pharmacy are profound. No longer simply the dispenser of prescriptions and the first point of contact for advice on minor ailments, perhaps in the future the pharmacist may be the manager of medicines in primary care teams, the prescriber of medication where licensed and competent, and even the controller of the medicine budget of the primary care organisation.

Issues for the pharmacy in the sector

1. What is the place of community and the clinical pharmacy in the digital world?
2. What are the implications for those training to be pharmacists?
3. As drug delivery systems and methods/technologies change (transdermal, implant, digitally monitored and genetic), how does the pharmacist add value?
4. How does the pharmacist become part of the out-of-hospital care team?
5. How does the pharmacist empower individuals in the community to move away from reliance on unnecessary and ineffective products?

PROFESSIONAL MULTICULTURALISM

Medicine, nursing and pharmacy represent only three of the many professional cultures involved with the provision of healthcare in the sector. The heritage also involves the heritage of

- Dentistry
- Optical services
- Physiotherapy
- Occupational therapy
- Dietetics
- Chiropody
- And others as the potential for the sector to care for people with specialist care needs leads to their delivery at home

In addition, the close relationships between the sector and other sectors of welfare provision such as social care, the voluntary sector, community and youth work, and other local authority services such as environmental health and housing have played an important part in the development of the primary healthcare sector and are likely to continue to be important for the sector's further development. Indeed as technology and demography drive change, so the historic boundaries in the welfare system seem less relevant to the current situation.

It is important to recognise that the heritage of each element is different but complementary to the heritage of the whole sector ([30] figure 1.2 p. 19 of *The Challenge for Primary Care*). Adding value to the matrix of cultures which characterise the primary care sector is the different emphasis that each puts on issues such as:

- Personal and continuing care
- Promoting personal autonomy
- Commercial and business interests
- The interest of the community versus the interests of the individual
- Personal responsibility
- Gatekeeping either to state resources or to other parts of the welfare system
- Democratic accountability

While the emphasis differ among all the groups involved, it is clear that the differences matter to many of those involved and underpin many of the attitudes, values and beliefs which affect relationships and performance in the sector.

The degree of cohesion between the cultures making up the sector has to be a major interest of primary care organisations, which, while reflecting on the values of what they have inherited from the past, must seek to deliver a new coherence within the sector if it is to adapt successfully to its future responsibilities.

The task for primary care organisations of coordinating such provision has been likened to playing tennis with a raspberry, but is perhaps seen better as creating an orchestra from a group of specialist musicians.

Rather than concentrating on the diversity of the cultural heritage and the fact that so many of the cultures relate to each other without much common ground, we need to emphasise their complementary nature. All the different groups and interests involved in the sector have contributed to the heritage of the sector and continue to contribute to its success – they all play their part in the "score". But just as different players will master their own instrument so too do different players in the primary care sector. The coordination and teamwork which distinguish a successful orchestra from an ordinary one are just as important in primary care. Too often players have failed to mould their efforts to the needs of the sector and the individuals it serves, and have been, as a result, less than effective team players.

REFLECTION

Chris (my father) had wanted to be a paediatric surgeon, but following a bout of TB successfully treated in 1943 he decided to become a GP. He joined Dr Elliott (see Chapter 1, Box 1.1) in 1946 and remained in the practice for the rest of his working life, initially as an "assistant" and then as a partner. The partnership was really a group of four single-handed GPs working across a scattered population of about 8000 people living in the Chiltern Hills between High Wycombe and Oxford. These were all dispensing doctors who started a pharmacy – (managed by Arthur Young for over thirty years), and worked with the community nurse Joyce and other local community nursing staff, but were otherwise professionally isolated. He visited all his patients at home when they were unable to come to surgery and in hospital – and the Shrubbery Maternity Unit. Initially, the work was tough: long hours in surgery from 8 am to 7:30 pm; a large number of home visits, frequently over ten per day; and the on-calls were onerous (he was on six nights per week and covered Tony, the nearest partner in Stokenchurch when he had his day and night off). The developments outlined earlier formed the backdrop to his career: he was a founder member of the RCGP; a friend of John Horder and Dame Annis Gillee; and he saw the introduction of the primary care team, health centre and GP training as a local course organiser. In his retirement in the 1980s many of the issues detailed earlier formed the scenery of our walks across the countryside. He was a firm believer in the value of the "medical model" but did not consider the NHS had got the design of primary care right. Local people needed the power and had to be equipped to cope with the responsibility to direct and control their health service, and for him, it was always their service. I know he was ashamed that poor quality care provision and inadequate performance by colleagues was not effectively tackled and I know he felt the RCGP and BMA's GP Committee (the General Medical Services Committee [GMSC] at that time) had become ineffective and ill equipped to lead the sector into the future. He was also very sceptical about political control of the NHS. He wanted it be independent with a long-term charter – like the BBC – and he wanted patients to take control.

REFERENCES

1. Starfield B. 1994. Is primary care essential? *Lancet* 344:1129–33.
2. Rivett G. 1998. *From Cradle to Grave*. Kings Fund, London.
3. Dawson B. 1918. The future of the medical profession (Cavendish Lecture). *Lancet* 2:83–5.
4. Ministry of Health, Consultative Council on Medical and Allied Services. 1920. Interim report on the future provision of medical and allied services (Chairman Lord Dawson). CMD 693. HMSO, London.
5. Beveridge W. 1942. *Social Insurance and Allied Services*. Para 428. HMSO, London.
6. Timmins N. 1995. *The Five Giants*. Harper Collins, London.
7. Ministry of Health. 1946. National Health Service Bill, summary of the proposed new service. CMD 6761. HMSO, London.
8. Ministry of Health. 1948. *National Health Service Patients Guides*. HMSO, London.
9. Collins JS. 1953. Group practice. *Lancet* 2:31–3; 611–15; 875–7.
10. Care Quality Commission. 2017. *The State of Care in General Practice 2014–2017*. CQC, London.
11. Hadfield SJ. 1953. Field survey of General Practice (1951–2). *BMJ* 2:683.

12. Taylor S. 1954. *Good General Practice: A Report on the Survey*. Nuffield Provincial Hospital Trust/Oxford University Press, London.
13. Ministry of Health. 1953. Report of the Ministry of Health for the year ending 31 December 1952, Part 1. CMD 8933. HMSO, London.
14. Royal College of General Practitioners. 1966. *Evidence of the Royal Commission of Medical Education: Report from General Practice, No. 5*. RCGP, London.
15. Gillie A. 1963. *The Field of Work of the Family Doctor*. HMSO, London.
16. Porritt report on the N.H.S. 1962. *BMJ* 2:1171.
17. Illich I. 1975. *Limits to Medicine: Medical Nemesis; The Expropriation of Health*. Penguin, London.
18. Department of Health. 1997. *The new NHS: Modern, dependable*. DoH White Paper, London.
19. Griffiths R. 1983. NHS management inquiry. *BMJ* 287:1391–4.
20. Committee on the Financial Aspects of Corporate Governance. 1992. *The financial aspects of corporate governance [Cadbury Report]*. Gee Professional Publishing, London.
21. NHS England. 2014. *Five Year Forward View*. NHSE, London.
22. NHS England. 2016. *General Practice Forward View*. NHSE, London.
23. British social attitudes survey. 2017. King's Fund Analysis 2.1.2018. https://www.kingsfund.org.uk/publications/public-satisfaction-nhs-social-care-2018.
24. King's Fund quarterly monitoring report June 2017. https://qmr.kingsfund.org.uk.2017/23.
25. House of Commons Health Committee. 2016. Primary care: Fourth report of session 2015–16. HC 408. www.parliament.uk/healthcare.
26. Tudor Hart. 2000. Commentary: Three decades of the Inverse care law. *BMJ*. 320(7226):18–19.
27. Abel-Smith B. 1982. *History of the Nursing Profession*. Heinemann, London.
28. Modi N. 2017. Attitudes of breastfeeding must change in UK. *Guardian*. August 1.8.2017.
29. Holloway SWF. 1991. *Royal Pharmaceutical Society of Great Britain. 1841–1991*. Pharmaceutical Press, London.
30. Starey N. 2003. *The Challenge for Primary Care*. Radcliffe Medical Press, Oxford. ISBN 1-85775-569-3.

4

The current situation in primary care: From analysis to interpretation

INTRODUCTION

Analysing any complex situation requires a systematic approach to considering all the factors involved and how they relate to each other. This is an iterative process in which interim results may need reanalysing as time and events move on. In medicine the analysis usually starts with listening to the patient's story or taking their history systematically; this is followed by close inspection or examining the patient overall and particularly any areas of concern; then tests or investigations follow in order to clarify or substantiate concerns. All these steps help establish a diagnosis, but once again this may be reviewed in an iterative fashion as further evidence emerges.

So, it is important that we listen to the story of the primary care sector – both its history, or heritage, as explained in Chapters 1, 2 and 3, and its experience of the current situation through its and our own eyes. Although rather subjective, individual stories have "added value" because they reflect how people feel about their current experience of the sector. In the last five years, I have visited over a hundred general practices as part of the Care Quality Commission (CQC) inspection programme [2], interviewed over two hundred healthcare practitioners on those visits and heard their stories along with those of patients visiting on the day of inspection. I then read, reviewed and considered reports on over 2000 inspections for quality assurance purposes and confirmed their ratings.

In addition in 2017, I walked the 640 miles of the South West Coast Path, from Minehead in Somerset to Poole in Dorset, and used this as an opportunity to talk to over a hundred people I met along the way about their experience of primary care services. Perhaps a fitter-than-average group and perhaps a little older than a random sample, but nevertheless a series of stories told over anything from a few minutes to a couple of days – unhurried and mostly uninterrupted. I found these conversations hugely important in helping me reflect on my own experience of the sector. A few highlights from the hundreds of rich stories and experiences which have informed this section and indeed the entire book.

- Brian (on the cliff's of the Lizard): "I'm doing this to show the back surgeon that he's wrong. I may not be back on my mountain bike yet, but he said I had to accept the reality that my back injury would mean a lifetime on painkillers and no more sport. I've managed five days walking so far, and I've just sent him a postcard. I don't want his pills and I'm determined to enjoy my life in my own way. I've been a council groundsman for forty years and I'm back there, but they have bought me a sit-down motor mower".
- Wendy: "I used to be a district nurse, but I just love the patients here [a GP practice]. I see the mums and babies, the youngsters, their parents and grandparents. I see the homeless and the frail, the rich and the poor – but they all come in for my help and I just love it. The best thing – celebrating one year off the fags with our postman. Oh, and taking a smear test from a woman whose sister had died from cancer and who had been unable to even come into the surgery for seven years and then it took me another five years to win her over. Happily the smear was fine".
- YG, who had been a senior executive in the healthcare industry (and had the most amazing toe'd walking shoes), had such insight into how commercial forces can get in the way of care, and how the healthcare industry can get in the way of an individual's happiness. Commercial interests come first in her work, whereas in the health service people try to put the patient's interest first. She had now left her job and was planning when she finished her walk to move into National Health Service (NHS) management.
- The GP partner who cried as she told me of her resignation from the partnership because she felt unable to care for her patients: The corporate support her partnership had brought in had introduced new systems and now expected the partners to be the duty doctors every day, with admin support, which meant filling the "book on the day" slots for the salaried staff to see. "I just can't do it. I don't see my patients, and it's not safe. My partners and I are all leaving. I don't want to be responsible for this shambles. We were a good stable partnership – a training practice and proud of the standard of care we provided. When two partners retired we really struggled to recruit new partners and ended up with two advanced nurse practitioners and an excellent salaried GP. When a further GP partner retired we knew we were in trouble and that was when we looked beyond the practice for management support. Our own practice manager has now left because she felt the culture and approach is no longer something she can support, and I am following her to be a salaried GP in her new practice".

A little more objective are some of the submissions to the recent 2015 House of Commons Health Select Committee's enquiry into primary care [1]. These submissions to this enquiry told the picture as they saw it – it was always from their own perspective and biased by their experience. The summary of the enquiry (Box 4.1) is really useful to our analysis. It brings together all the stories, or evidence, it heard and provides an authoritative report. However, the enquiry was established to consider "the extent to which the primary care sector is meeting the needs of the population" and in this it falls someway short. Because, by failing to weigh and balance all the perspectives involved in the sector and to systematically address the needs of the population alongside the extent to which the sector is currently meeting them, or could potentially meet them, the enquiry's findings are weakened.

BOX 4.1: House of Commons Select Committee Enquiry into Primary Care 2015–2016

The following is a summary of the committee's findings:

SUMMARY

Primary care is the bedrock of the National Health Service and the setting for ninety percent of all NHS patient contacts. It is highly valued by the public but is under unprecedented strain and struggling to keep pace with relentlessly rising demand. The traditional model of ten-minute appointments with general practitioners no longer allows them to provide the best possible care for patients living with increasingly complex long-term conditions.

The difficulty in accessing primary care is a serious concern for many patients, especially for those who work during the week. We believe that it is vital that patients have timely access to primary care services. This includes both access to urgent appointments and the ability to book routine appointments in advance.

During the course of this inquiry we heard many examples of innovative practice which give cause for optimism that patients' access to and experience of primary care can be improved. The priority for government should be to train, develop and retain not only more GPs but wider multi-disciplinary teams working within a more integrated system of care. Patients would also benefit from the better use of technology to assist communication with and between their clinicians. There is a pressing need to improve continuity and safety through the use of electronic patient records which can be shared, with their consent, wherever people access their care.

In line with the recommendations of the Primary Care Workforce Commission, multi-disciplinary teams can harness the skills not only of GPs but physiotherapists, practice nurses, pharmacists, mental health workers and physician associates. We support the Commission's vision of teams of professionals using their skills to meet the needs of patients much earlier in their journey through the NHS. This would allow GPs to concentrate on those aspects of care that only they can provide. We expect GP leaders to be at the forefront of the development of multi-disciplinary teams.

Patients need more health professionals from a range of disciplines to choose careers in primary care. Existing medical education does not encourage graduates to do so and greater attention must be paid to the needs of patients in designing training pathways and incentives across the entire NHS workforce. It is far from certain that sufficient numbers of GPs and nurses will be available to build new teams and improve patient access. Much greater efforts to recruit, train and retain the primary care workforce will be necessary if the vision of the Primary Care Workforce Commission is to be achieved.

The government made a manifesto commitment to seven day access to services but further clarification is needed about how this commitment is to be implemented and resourced, especially in light of the workforce shortfall.

Improving access to primary care is a welcome goal, but practical application of the seven day policy should be locally designed, led by the evidence and take account of local recruitment challenges. The policy must also focus on the continuity of patient care and avoid reducing the capacity of weekday services as well as urgent out of hours primary care cover. Although difficulty in accessing general practice continues to frustrate patients, GPs consistently receive highly positive patient satisfaction ratings. Healthwatch England pointed out that service users are reluctant to criticise their doctors and caution that the figures may mask deep-seated concerns about quality and standards.

We heard worrying evidence about the longstanding variation in quality across primary care. The Care Quality Commission has highlighted very poor standards of care among a small proportion of practices and has developed a mechanism to close those which put their patients at risk and to follow up necessary improvements in others.

We welcome the benefits which CQC inspection has brought for patients and we urge the Royal College of General Practitioners and the British Medical Association to work constructively with the CQC to protect the public from failing practices and to help to turn around underperforming practices. At the same time, NHS England, the CQC, the General Medical Council and Local Education and Training Boards must work together to reduce bureaucracy and unnecessary duplication, so that time which should be devoted to patient care is not eroded by an excessive bureaucratic burden.

Despite the rising demand for services and a consensus on the value of primary care, its funding has fallen behind as a share of the overall NHS budget. The five-year funding settlement provides only a very limited uplift in expenditure on primary care. We believe that it should receive a larger proportion of overall NHS spending in order to improve access and services for patients.

GAPS

Among the many excellent submissions that the committee heard there were a few omissions which would have helped them move beyond simply hearing the stories and move into the territory of systematic enquiry through which, in medicine, we question the storyteller to tease out further issues of importance. In this instance, these issues would have included:

1. The suitability of current business models through which care is organised and delivered in the sector.
2. The strength or weaknesses of the relationships between the care providers making up the teams caring for individual people in the sector.
3. The extent to which the health priorities of the community are receiving due attention in the sector.
4. The extent to which the sector is "fit for purpose" and "fit for the future" as the digital context flowers.
5. The degree to which the relationship between citizens and care providers has evolved during the time of the NHS to reflect the differing views of generations.
6. The boundary between the care that citizens ought to take personal responsibility for and that which the NHS should provide for them.
7. The value of the lifelong medical record and any continuing relationship with care providers over time – biographical care, as opposed to episodic care, whether or not informed by personal medical records.
8. The value of "gatekeeping" as a regulator of access to services beyond the sector as compared to a care coordinator approach.
9. The degree to which the sector is effectively integrating care to meet the needs of the population, including links between general practice, general dentistry, ophthalmic services, community pharmacy, community nursing services, health visiting, social services, occupational health, physiotherapy, audiology, chiropody and other specialist services that can be effectively delivered to support people in their own home.
10. The extent the current contracting mechanisms, through which the provision of care is organised, is fit for purpose. Is the current general medical services (GMS)/ personal medical services (PMS)/alternative provider medical services (APMS) national contracting approach to general practice complementing or conflicting with the frameworks underpinning other services, such as those provided in the hospital sector and those in community pharmacy and optical services?
11. Are the corporate and clinical governance systems in the sector sufficiently robust, open and trustworthy?
12. Are the current medicine supply arrangements through dispensing and community pharmacy services either in retail or digital environments appropriate?
13. Is the capitalisation of the sector enabling the provision of appropriate services in appropriate facilities?
14. Are the relationships between different services (among walk-in centres, GP out-of-hours services, GP hub services, GP practices, community nursing services, ambulance accident and emergency [A&E], and specialist services for

example) sufficiently clear and coordinated to ensure members of the public receive seamless care? Is coordination helped or hindered by the accessibility of individuals' health records?

These concerns – and I am sure there are others – require answers through a process of "intrusive enquiry". But in the absence of that – and there is nobody undertaking it – inspection or systematic and targeted examination can help us move towards analysis. We will then need to use some analytical tools to help us move towards interpretation of our findings.

For the first time in the history of the NHS we have recently had a systematic, comprehensive inspection programme in English general practice supplemented by the inspection of other providers in the primary care sector, such as out-of-hours providers, walk-in centres, general dental practice, NHS 111 services and those providing online digital services to the community. This programme, developed and run by the Care Quality Commission [2], provides a great deal of information about the performance of the sector through a quality assured reporting system which has rated all GP practices against an agreed template and which goes some way to replacing "subjective review" with "objective inspection". I have personally visited over seventy inspections and been involved with reading reporting and agreeing ratings for over two thousand of the seven thousand reports. Collectively this body of work celebrates the performance of general practice and the primary care sector as the best performing care sector of those have been inspected and rated anywhere in the world. The programme has been delivered in the face of sometimes vituperative opposition from some stakeholders, who tried unsuccessfully to disrupt the programme, and in sometimes distressing circumstances where stressed practices and practitioners found the process of inspection difficult to endure. Nevertheless, the programme is complete and we owe it to all those who were inspected to make sure that the results are respected, valued and used to contribute to the necessary analysis that this chapter offers. The CQC programme report [2] is clear in highlighting the fact that the key determinants of performance include leadership and safe systems, that staffing and access arrangements are currently stressed and that the process of "special measures" to address inadequacy can improve the quality of care patients receive. It is not the purpose of the CQC to offer the services of a quality improvement agency – it is a regulator– or to make recommendations about any improvements or developments which are required. But its evidence can and should be used as a support for our analysis, and the following is a brief description of how the CQC findings can help us interpret the findings of inspection.

The lack of any systematic approach to *quality improvement* in the sector and of anybody with responsibility for it has to be of concern – especially when the sector is so central to the delivery of the NHS purpose.

LESSONS FROM THE CQC INSPECTION PROGRAMME

The CQC inspection programme [2] in English primary care successfully completed the first-ever comprehensive inspection of all English general practices, published its results at both the individual practice level and as an overall programme report, and deserves credit for completing this in the face of vituperative and well-coordinated negativism. However, I believe CQC can and should offer more analysis of the challenges the sector is facing and offer more colour to the vision of the future that general practice and other providers involved in the primary care sector might evolve into.

I offer eleven lessons to start the task of reinvigorating the sector to be fit for the future and which can add the "targeted" examination element to this chapter's analysis section.

1. The sector is currently being *stressed* by demographic and economic forces, while technological developments mean it could provide an even greater proportion of the care its patients need. But it does not have the capacity – the workforce, the infrastructure or the resources – to achieve this in any systematic, quality assured way which can be trusted. This *capacity/capability* mismatch is a particular stressor to the predominant organisational form "professional partnership", which is ill-suited to meet the needs of modern society (i.e. power sharing, openness and accountability and for greater empowerment of service users) and it is also ill-suited to the needs and preferences of modern professional life (i.e. greater flexibility, a better work–life balance and more family friendly arrangements). In response to these *stressors* the resilience of the sector is remarkable, but weaker providers in areas where the stresses are greatest, such as those of greatest deprivation or demographic extremes, are too often failing, which only makes the pressure more extreme on neighbouring practices and other providers making up the local health economy. I call this the *governance* challenge because its essence is the weakness of the arrangements that make it safe for us all – users, providers and the wider community – to trust the sector.

   Access is another stressor which has divided practices during the inspection programme. On the whole, "good" and "outstanding" practices are currently *thriving despite rising demand* from the population for better access to care. They have adapted telephone arrangements, extended surgery sessions and time per consultation, organised "hub" arrangements in localities to provide seven-day appointments – basically, "sweated the asset". In contrast many "requiring improvement" or "inadequate" practices are *drowning in demand*. Clinicians are working really hard, but in organisations that are not coping are often not fit for purpose because they are so busy meeting the demands from their patients that they cannot see the organisations' needs. The weakness is often one of management and leadership – they are fighting fire with buckets instead of foam.

2. But we should move beyond this – to understand the reasons leading to rising demand and the stresses it causes. Later, we shall return to this issue when we analyse or use "tests and investigations" to get underneath the issues and in later chapters when we use the tools of systems theory and lateral thinking to liberate our minds to possible solutions. If form is to follow function, then having realised that transformation is happening we should ensure we understand and are equipped to address the functions before we leap to form.

BL was a well-respected local practice in Westhampton until three GP retirements a few years ago and an influx of patients from a new housing development meant patient access became a thorny issue and the results of their patient survey went into decline. Skill substitution, triage and "book on the day" care coordinators and care managers all helped a bit, but everyone was too busy so "growth and underinvestment" was the system archetype being played out (see Chapter 5) even bringing an external "support agency" did not prevent the practice being rated inadequate. This *vicious cycle* of decline requires "special measures" and even then the CQC's experience has been that special measures are often not enough to provide for a resilient and sustainable future.

CR is a practice with over 12,000 patients in a deprived inner London borough with over eighty percent from black or ethnic minority backgrounds and it has recently "hosted" patients from a practice which closed. It is a training practice and has a broad skill mix in its workforce. Despite huge challenges, this practice is thriving. The leadership from the management and partners is dynamic and committed. This mindset (see Chapter 5), a can-do approach permeating the whole team and was the reason it was able to recruit despite being in an area where others found it difficult and helped them drive a *virtuous cycle* of learning and improvement. I call this the dynamic and proactive *leadership* challenge. Because of a lack of focus and investment in leadership in the sector throughout the seventy years of NHS Mk 1, we have inherited a situation where performance is driven by reaction to circumstance rather than driven by the needs of the local population. I call this reactive management and leadership approach.

3. Such a lack of *cohesion* and *planning* to meet the needs of local populations has meant that care is too often disorganised and uncoordinated. In the early years of the NHS, resources in the community were sparse, but over time (see Chapter 2) effective primary care teams, comprising district nurses, health visitors, social workers, GPs ,and sometimes other local professionals such as school nurses, worked together and developed effective ways of coordinating care. Even in these periods, when the Family Practitioner Committee (FPC) and Family Health Service Authority (FHSA) had responsibility for administering the sector, there was little coordination with social care providers, and the focus was predominantly on doctoring and nursing – healthcare rather than welfare. Unfortunately, the CQC inspection programme has found *few* examples of effective coordination in the sector at the present time, and evidence of any planned approach to ensuring cohesion and effective provision across organisational boundaries is also largely lacking. It has sometimes seemed like a deliberate policy to fragment primary care has been followed – district nurses into area teams, health visitors into children's centres, midwives into outreach teams, social workers having generic area caseloads. All at a time when the need is for the NHS to focus on delivering efficient, coordinated planned care within its allocated budget rather than circling the wagons, protecting budget boundaries and making short-sighted finance-driven decisions to the detriment of its population's health needs and its own effectiveness. For the

want of an effective commissioner or an efficient coordinator of the primary care sector, we have developed a *disintegrated* service.

The practice in Baston used to have community nurses and its health visitor based in the building. Its counsellor, community psychiatric nurse (CPN), social worker, specialist nurses, midwife and physio all visited for sessions in the surgery, and they all met either informally around individual care needs or more formally for care planning meetings. On a recent CQC inspection the practice's safeguarding lead discussed the fact that in recent times they never met the health visitor – they communicated by phone or fax. She also felt that antenatal liaison with the midwife had become more distant to the extent that the GPs had little involvement with pregnancy or the puerperium. A recent issue with postnatal depression and domestic abuse had raised safeguarding concerns in her mind, but the vital liaison discussions with those involved were really difficult to organise. She had read and reflected on a recent "serious case review" into a child's death and realised that one of its central recommendations about communications and inter-agency cooperation could apply in, and need to be addressed, in her local area as well.

4. Current arrangements for *contracting* for services in the sector are historic legacies from NHS Mk 1 and are no longer fit for purpose in the modern digital world. The national GMS and PMS contracts provide little incentive for practices to systematically address local health needs and support the local health economy. For example, because GP partners are self-employed independent contractors, if they invest in their practices to provide additional services or staff, practice profitability often falls and their take-home pay reduces. Many practices have seen such significant reductions in partners' take-home pay that their ability to retire and recruit new partners is compromised. Many trained GPs would rather work as a salaried doctor or as a locum than set sail on a career as a partner. Although the development of the PMS contract was an attempt to provide some local flexibility to address service needs and reward investment, it has frequently failed to meet this aspiration, at least partly because investment in commissioning skills in the sector is underdeveloped. National contract negotiations by one stakeholder, the British Medical Association, inevitably focus on the view it sees (i.e. the medical view of the world), whereas the needs of the population and sector for healthcare and more broadly welfare are much broader and require an approach to agreement between providers and commissioners, which drives transformation of the sector rather than preserves the status quo. During the CQC inspection programme, there were many examples of practices which had broken out of the medical model paradigm, in recognition of the need to contribute to a healthy community. But they had to do much of this work pro bono. There were also too many practices that had retreated, licking their wounds from the frontline, recognising that the historic way to maximise profits in general practice has been to reduce overheads, reduce investment and maximise registrations. Rather there is a need for a framework of local contracting for the services the local community needs, a framework which supports challenge to the inverse care law [3] so that investment is in

proportion to the needs of the community rather than inversely proportional to it. Of course, a simple weighting of resources to need using a weighting scale such a deprivation factor will be neither politically or socially acceptable, but at least it would move us towards the systematic challenge required.

5. There are brilliant examples of the sector providing effective, coordinated care to meet the needs of the *frail elderly*, but these are isolated pixels in a picture of huge unmet need, where families struggle to care for isolated relatives often miles away, without effective support and feel guilty when they fail; and where feelings of loneliness and worthlessness are endemic. In this world where "Granny farming" into care homes is regarded as the best option because family and community support has become rudimentary and fragmented by economic and social forces; where the political imperative is to win votes at the next election rather than to build a community fit to care for its heritage and its heroes. In this world there is a need for a more systematic, sympathetic and coordinated programme to identify and describe, design and provide care for this vulnerable group – which may well include all of us in future years – in a way which preserves dignity and values experience. The CQC has seen brilliant work to support carers, ensure the needs of the most vulnerable are met in the community rather than in the revolving door of the A&E department and which support the community to care. But there is no mechanism, no design feature, no incentive for the pixels so spread [8]. The local NHS needs to support carers and the care homes they work in with training and support, management, and clinical input. The CQC also needs to ensure that its inspections support work across the sector boundaries rather than reinforcing artificial boundaries.

Red practice had implemented a multidisciplinary team approach (doctor nurses, physio and occupational therapy, their clinical pharmacist and care coordinator) to caring for the frail elderly with a "virtual ward". But then the area was a popular retirement destination and now thirty years on it faced eighteen percent of its patient list being over eighty-five. It has redesigned the service, with a multidisciplinary team approach to the care of those with frailty either in their own home or in residential care. The practice developed care plans and built good relationships with the local community – the council, churches, schools and the voluntary sector were working with the practice to make their area a safer place to be frail.

Blue practice also reported that caring for the frail elderly was a big issue. Eighty percent of its home visiting was to the elderly, some of its care homes were asking for visits almost every day, the attached staff members were declining to visit nursing and residential care homes as they felt they were not adequately resourced for the workload. They were following a "shifting the burden" approach (see Chapter 5). CQC should become a proponent of mechanisms through which both the inverse care law and the rule of halves are challenged [3].

6. CQC has mainly seen "good" *safeguarding systems* in the great majority of its inspections, but this has to be seen against the agreed "base camp" benchmark of appropriate training, identified leadership, available information about the local

safeguarding system and participation in local arrangements by the provision of reports ([4]: *Intercollegiate guidance*). Really excellent work in the safeguarding system – the proactive identification of the vulnerable through relationships which they trust; focussed systems to support the vulnerable; participation as "representatives and advocates" at case conferences and core group meetings; effective liaison with social services and health visiting; participation in enquiries and reviews; and above all effective engagement with teams supporting and ensuring the safety of the most vulnerable – is seldom seen but desperately needed.

Because these elements are absent from the design of the sector. Serious case reviews involving child victims such as Maria Caldwell, Rikki Neave and Victoria Climbie have all pointed to gaps in the system protecting vulnerable children. But the response from general practice and the wider primary care sector has been deafening in its silence. Other vulnerable people – the frail elderly, those with learning disabilities, and those experiencing domestic violence, abused by genital mutilation, subject to domestic slavery or trafficked into prostitution – fare no better. Surely it must be the hallmark of a caring society and a testament to the founding fathers of the modern welfare state that it finally becomes designed to protect the weak and surely if general practitioners are trained to see themselves as "the patient's agent" then this must include being proactive in support of those needing safeguarding.

Too often there seems to be a mindset in general practices that these safeguarding issues are peripheral to them. The lead agency is social services and they sometimes marginalise practices – their case conferences are impossible to get to, always during surgery time and miles away, and practices don't feel they are valued partners. This mindset's narrow vision of their role being to identify and refer rather than to analyse and support decision making is unfortunate. It thrives where practices focus on the demands of the worried well to the detriment of the vulnerable and the sick. CQC has done the country a great service by inspecting the sector and holding a mirror up to each and every organisation it has inspected. Now is the time for the sector to learn lessons and ensure the NHS Mk 2 "digital" world moves beyond "base camp", to accept that its responsibility is to challenge this mindset and ensure it is designed to protect the weak. Use of digital technology to join case conferences by Skype for example has to be encouraged.

CH was an inner-city practice. The GPs explained they had reviewed their safeguarding procedures and had recognised the need to improve safeguarding. In response, they carried out a number of searches on the patient database to identify patients who may be vulnerable. To date they have ensured that staff members were alerted to the risks of 100 children. Within this they had identified children who were on the child protection register, children in need, those who had social service involvement and those in care. In addition, they had trained staff and discussed the issues of vulnerability each month in their customer care meeting to ensure all staff could prioritise these cases when they visited the practice. They had set up a safeguarding team in the practice consisting of two GPs, a healthcare assistant and two administration staff to ensure that they continued to identify and monitor children and adults at risk of abuse.

7. *Learning organisations* [5] are those which understand the environment they live in and develop their plans as a result of learning from their experience of that environment. While the CQC inspection programme has looked at elements of the "anatomy" of the learning system in primary care. It has not looked beyond the anatomy to inspect the "physiology" of the system – the way it responds and the outcomes of that response. While reviewing complaints, considering significant events and performing staff appraisals are all happening in the great majority of provider practices and organisations, they are seen as isolated elements rather than joined together as part of a learning system driving improvement.

GH practice saw itself as a *learning organisation*. It celebrated significant events and complaints as opportunities to learn and improve. The recent unexpected death of a young man, Mustafa, registered with the practice, was an example. He had died at aged twenty-six from cardiomyopathy. The practice met with the pathologist to discuss the implications, visited the gym where Mustafa had been taken ill, talked to the paramedics who had been called out and taken Mustafa to hospital, and arranged a review meeting with Mustafa's family and everyone who had been involved. The practice's learning included working with the gym to screen other apparently fit young men, fundraising with the ambulance trust to buy and then train volunteers to use defibrillators, and also discussing with Mustafa's imam the issues raised by first-cousin marriage, including consanguinity and the increased risk of inherited disease which it involves.

From the start of the NHS there has been no attempt to encourage sector leadership, to systematically value quality improvement and to drive out poor practice. Until CQC tackled areas of poor performance that it found on inspection, these failings were too often ignored. Often they were known about quite widely but allowed to fester for years without being effectively tackled. This has led to poor care – harming people's health, risking their future and wasting money. This has been uncomfortable territory for CQC to tackle and the answer is beyond CQCs remit and purpose. NHS improvement has no mandate in primary care and nor does any other organisation. Unfortunately, there is little in the way of sector expertise to call on to tackle this void. CQC's "special measures" teams, drawn from the Royal College of General Practitioners (RCGP) and local commissioners, must catalyse a more systematic and sustainable systemic approach to ensuring the sector learns from experience to improve the quality of care it provides.

8. One of the effects of the variety of contracting arrangements for primary care services within the NHS has been a *lack of coordination* between providers in the sector. General practice used to be responsible for the medical care of registered patients twenty-four hours a day, seven days a week, and this remained the case until the development of GP cooperative (out-of-hours) arrangements in the mid-1990s. Removing the overall responsibility of GPs has led to the emergence of a range of alternative providers – walk-in centres, corporate out-of-hours providers, minor injury centres, hubs, nurse- and paramedic-led clinics and GPs at the front end of A&E, NHS direct, and now

NHS 111 – all developed with the best of intentions to deal with the demand from the public for access and of course they have provided more choice for consumers of healthcare. But none of them were planned and coordinated to ensure safe and effective care based on a comprehensive, lifelong clinical record of people's health. Too many people still end up in A&E when they don't need to. They go there because they struggle to navigate this complicated system, particularly when they are vulnerable as a result of pain, sickness or anxiety. The CQC inspection programme has looked at all the plethora of providers and found much good practice within each organisation, but little evidence of cohesive working between providers and little evidence of effective public engagement to ensure appropriate design to meet the needs of the community. Too many services have been commissioned from large corporate providers on grounds of cost at the expense of quality. Too many GP-led out-of-hours social enterprises have succumbed to lack of support from local clinicians, who have prohibitive insurance costs and heavy daytime pressures to overcome to offer support by working extra time as clinicians. In addition many feel that they would be supporting a contracting framework which seeks to promote economies of scale beyond what clinicians feel appropriate – clinical cover too thin on the ground to provide safe care for the community. This is a picture of *disintegration*, in some areas frankly dangerous disintegration. Communities deserve better and we have a responsibility to design and deliver it.

Somershire's GP out-of-hours service is provided by a national group, which also provides walk-in centres and minor injury units, has taken over several failing practices and also provides call-centre services. In the past the GP co-op staffed eight local centres at times of high demand and kept four centres working through the night. The new corporate provider has struggled to recruit staff, and frequently there has only been one "floating" care with GP and driver for the whole county. *The vicious cycle of decline again.*

In another area despite a very scattered and difficult-to-reach population, innovative recruitment approaches and high-quality local leadership have supported an "outstanding" service where integration with other services in the local health economy, a driven approach to individual and organisational learning, and a determination to continuously improve quality have helped to retain high staffing levels and strong support from local general practice. *The virtuous cycle of quality improvement again.*

9. The template for inspections used by CQC inspection teams has been developed following consultation and is acknowledged to be the most comprehensive, systematic tool ever applied as a quality assurance mechanism in the sector. Nevertheless the tool has a few important blind spots which need highlighting. Just as CQC has shone its spotlight into areas which have for too long been shielded from view, so too these are areas that require more attention in NHS Mark 2. First, it is clear that there are a group of key national priorities which the government requires the NHS to focus on, but the NHS has thus far been unable to design an effective delivery framework. Smoking, cancer, obesity, dementia, diabetes, adolescent mental health and addiction have all been widely discussed as key priorities for several years. But while the sector has

played an effective role in reducing the burden caused by smoking, improving the care of patients with diabetes and improving outcomes for people who develop cancer, there is still considerable room for improvement. As a result there is too great a range of patient experience when they are faced with these issues. The lack of any systematic programme in these key areas has led to both virtuous and vicious circles developing in isolation.

The Care Quality Commission has to become more involved as an agent supporting change through quality improvement. Without greater focus in the sector there will inevitably be more harm, early deaths and widespread distress because effective holistic approaches to each of these national priority issues requires a generalist, primary care engaged programme. The absence of responsibility being assigned to any agency for this black hole cannot excuse the current failure to address it. Just as the reduction in cervical cancer deaths and the reduction in hospital admissions for diabetes [6] are not entirely due to primary care's efforts – but those efforts have been important – so coordinated efforts by the sector are needed in the other key areas. CQC has found much good care for people with long-term conditions where incentivised through the Quality and Outcomes Framework (QOF), but this systematic approach needs to be broadened to the other key national priority areas and other long-term conditions which have been overshadowed for too long by the QOF. Multiple sclerosis, macular degeneration, psoriasis, osteoarthritis and hearing loss appear on every GPs list, but none receive the kind of systematic care sufferers deserve and the CQC's inspection methodology allows this to continue because it prioritises and focusses attention on those conditions rewarded by QOF arrangements rather than other "forgotten" conditions.

10. *Looking at things differently.* The mandate CQC has been given by the government and has required it to inspect the safety and quality of care provided, but of course inspection of safety and quality has highlighted and hopefully clarified underlying issues which require attention if the health of the population is to be promoted. With more care being provided in the *home-based* arena, because it can be, and because national economic circumstance is promoting it, then attention needs to be paid to these underlying issues. The history of the NHS [13] is one of ever-increasing demands being made by the population on a service which has consumed an ever-increasing amount of money. But this is not unique to the NHS. All healthcare systems in the developed world share this experience, and when times are tough, then budgets are squeezed and the weakest are squeezed most. The analogy of us driving a Morris Minor when we need a Tesla comes to mind. When inspecting the 7000 English general practices the CQC did sometimes come across examples where practices had taken a radically different approach, where by employing a consistent set of policies designed to reduce demand on the NHS they had been able to reduce the cost of providing the service, liberating and *empowering* patients to take more control over their own health and well-being, sharing decision making with them and supporting them to be "active partners".

The OD practice in a market town in Dorset was established about twenty years ago and has followed a strategy of empowering patients to take control of their own health through programmes of education, supported decision making, active participation in individual and group health promotion. and disease prevention. Strong relationships between clinicians, staff and patients with a policy framework promoting delegated responsibility and investment in people as well as facilities, for example special screens to enhance vision and special "anti-infective" paint. The result was a folder presented to the CQC team detailing the practice's seventeen-year experience of reducing resource utilisation – reduced consulting rates, reduced prescribing, reduced hospital referral rates, outpatient attendance and A&E visits. This is a small practice but it shows what can be achieved when the prevalent mindset of dependency and the shifting-the-burden archetype (Chapter 5) are challenged.

11. Another area which is highlighted by reflection about CQC's inspection programme of English general practice is the issue of whether the *governance* arrangements remain fit for purpose in NHS Mark 2. I have already raised some concerns about partnership as an appropriate business model and the medical model [21] as an appropriate power holder. But what would be better? The current model has stood the test of time and is widely trusted? Evidence from New Zealand and elsewhere suggests that the new models of care and Vanguard arrangements being trialled in England under the umbrella of the *Five Year Forward View* [7] may help improve the effectiveness and efficiency of care in the sector, but that the APMS approach to privatisation of largely underperforming providers is frequently ineffective and sometimes simply a waste of resources, with inadequate performance failing to improve in a sustainable way, despite considerable investment through *special measures.*

A new approach to governance in the sector is required, and it needs to build on historic success rather than pickle it. It needs to balance openness and transparency with *trust* (see Chapter 1), respect and confidentiality; it needs to ensure that it is safe for people to trust the organisation with their health and with their life; that it is safe for clinicians and support staff to trust the organisation with their careers; and that it promotes safer communities and the welfare of all parts of those communities; that it works "by design" to make the local health economy more efficient and more effective. In the NHS Mk 1 it was trust which glued the doctor–patient relationship and underpinned the reputation of general practice as the foundation of the NHS. In NHS Mk 2 a new approach is needed to ensure that it remains safe for people who use the service, staff and the broader community to *trust* the service [8] – *Cornwall for example.* It is not just general practice – the whole of the primary care sector – or the out-of-hospital sector to ensure it becomes fit for purpose in the digital age.

Primary care in the digital age requires a new governance framework [9]. It is already apparent from early CQC inspections of digital providers that there are some risks associated with the current service models [9]:

- Segmentation – by cherry picking one or more sections of the population rather than respecting the NHS's social compact – paid for by the whole community and available to everyone.
- Lack of appropriately comprehensive health records being shared between digital providers and the NHS, such as with GPs.

- Weak safety netting to protect children and the vulnerable from exploitation.
- Distortion of "best prescribing" practice by being customer/demand led, antibiotics for example.
- Clinical staff who have been trained to provide biographical care as GPs and community pharmacists for example, now finding the digital sector is largely providing "episodic" care.

What would seem to be required is the absorption of the benefits of the digital approach to home-based healthcare, including ease and speed of consultation, convenience and confidentiality, but within a framework which also supports biographical care, that is care based on a long-term relationship when that it more appropriate. This is a subject we shall return to towards the end of the book.

INTERPRETATION

The next part of this book, starting from the end of this chapter, is concerned with using tools to interpret what is going on in the primary care sector. These tools – analogous to investigations in the medical world – challenge the *initial, tentative* diagnosis reached at the point where the story has been gathered and the sector been examined, in this case by CQC and the House of Commons Select Committee.

Before moving on to consider these tools of interpretation, a short time for reflection is always called for, just as with a patient it makes sense to ask "Does what the history and examination tell me, make sense?" In this case we shall consider whether our analysis fits the *context or circumstances* that the sector exists in. The tool we shall use to support this reflection is a PEST analysis [10] where we consider external forces affecting the development of the sector within four dimensions: the political forces operating in what is a highly politicised healthcare system; the economic forces operating to affect development; the sociocultural forces affecting the operation and development of the sector; and the technological changes and developments that are driving change.

POLITICAL FORCES

Looking at health through the lens of political determinants means analysing how different power constellations, institutions, processes, interests and ideological positions affect health within different political systems and cultures and at different levels of governance [11]. In focusing on the political forces affecting the primary care sector:

- At the global level where the rise of populism (rebellion against the neoliberal political establishment), the focus on globalisation (global capital, global corporations and global healthcare) and the rise of sustainability (fossil fuels, recycling and rising sea levels) are only glimpses of the tectonic plates within which the sector is evolving.

- At the national government level where, if politics is the exercise of power, the election cycle remains in conflict with the biographical, long-term relationship cultural aspects of the primary care sector's heritage. However, as our two major political parties evolve from their roots in libertarianism or egalitarianism to reflect the populist and enfranchised Britain of our post-industrial and post-family society, so the reality of the shift in public attitudes towards the NHS is thrown into relief. With the decline in confidence in the NHS [12], the intergenerational tensions and demographic pressures are dictating that the NHS's founding social compact, cradle to grave, and so on [13], could become unsustainable. More sticking plaster: a few more billions to get the service through the next election without trouble is not a credible solution. Without suggesting that our current political parties are overdue, a realignment to cope with Brexit and populism or that the NHS is due a realignment to cope with the digital world and the social transformation that has occurred since the service was established in 1946, it is hard to see how a way forward can be fashioned. But no doubt all will become clear in the near future.
- At the institutional level where decision-making power (royal colleges, unions and universities for example) has been concentrated in NHS Mk 1. Governance of the primary care sector by institutional influence is now being challenged by the rise of devolved power (such as clinical commissioning) and the decline of institutional power (examples such as "Care in the Community" and declining trade union membership come to mind). Similarly, the increasing importance of social media and digitally organised non-institutions, like crowd funding and "just giving", requires a devolved or distributed decision-making approach and a system of governance reflecting this process of deinstitutionalisation.
- Similarly at the professional (tribal) level, at the practice level and at the community level, the historic structural norms are being moulded and are responding to the same political forces. In the digital world of our present and our future, the relationship between the user and the provider of healthcare – in essence the power balance between them – has shifted. No longer is the power with the provider (i.e. the professional, the practice or the pharmacy, or the community staff); it has shifted towards the client/patient/user. The governance arrangements which promote trust and confidence [12] in these relationships ought to reflect the changing times.

ECONOMIC ISSUES

If economics is the study of how resources are used and health economics [15] involves maximising the output the NHS gets for its inputs (cost effectiveness and clinical effectiveness), then it is clear that the economic issues influencing the development of the primary care sector are not solely restricted to the financial allocation it receives each year from the exchequer. However, the resources do matter and the plans to invest in general practice outlined in the *GP Forward View* [22] – a fourteen percent increase in funding at a time when the rest of the NHS is receiving eight percent – offers some hope at the end of a long dark tunnel where

- Recruitment and retention of clinical staff is difficult and morale among GPs is low [14].
- Investment in the public sector has been constrained during recent years as part of government policy to address the national financial deficit.
- Workload in the sector has been increasing as a result of demographic pressures (see later) and continuing pressure elsewhere in the health and social care sectors.
- Cost pressures in the sector from professional costs, incremental wage growth and infrastructure costs have pressurised profitability, which is what the small business owners and self-employed independent contractors receive as income.
- At the global level the economic issues moulding the sector will include the migration of human resources to staff the sector, and the effect of withdrawal from the European Union, alongside government plans for additional clinical staff in the sector presumably as a result of migration from overseas.
- The health industry lives in a global market, that is, pharmaceutical companies are multinational, people travel and disease goes with them (flu pandemics and Ebola migrate as fast as airplanes travel).
- Healthcare systems around the world share their learning [20], the analysis shows many common problems, but highlights how well the NHS continues to perform overall in its use of resources and population coverage.
- At the national level NHS economics reflect government policy. In recent years this has meant years of constraint when the resources allocated have not kept pace with NHS inflation.
- While at the NHS management level the allocation of resources to primary care has had to follow historic precedence and take second place to dealing with acute hospital deficits.
- Within the primary care sector community pharmacy, ophthalmology and dentistry have been stressed by economic forces as much as general medical practice, and have seen reconfiguration and corporatisation as a consequence.

SOCIAL FACTORS

Our analysis must also be informed by the influence of social and cultural issues as they affect the sector:

- At the global level, world population growth and migration are important, but so too are the influences of widespread access to education and development opportunities in the developing world whose rate of economic growth is transforming social and cultural expectations.
- The primary care sector in Great Britain has thrived in a world of rapid social change during its first seventy years. Many issues are global but the ones we need to consider in our analysis include:
  - Changing family structures. Smaller families and delayed parenthood as a result of economic forces and the emancipation and employment opportunities for women have perhaps paradoxically led to greater reliance on the NHS. Parents have less informal healthcare advice from their families available close by and everyone has a mobile phone. However,

there are groups in our society with very different family norms, for example arranged marriage and first-cousin marriage are common in some Asian groups and single parenting with absent fathers is a feature in many parts of the country.

- Changing employment patterns. It's not just that we all change jobs several times in our careers, but we are less likely to work full time, we take more career breaks and retire at a younger age – so we have more leisure time.
- Changing housing arrangements. Not just an expectation of home ownership but also multigenerational occupancy – granny flats, young people living at home for longer, and intergenerational tensions resulting from different perspectives on wealth transfer, disposable income, holidays and savings.

- What is accepted behaviour has also been changing in recent years. Drink-driving and seat-belt wearing, smoking in public, gun and knife crime and gang culture are all issues affecting the primary care sector, either because of their effect on sickness or attitudes to healthcare.
- Of all the changing social forces, the rise in life expectancy and particularly the rise in the number of the frail elderly, the numbers living with dementia and the costs of social care have demanded greatest attention and been subject to most interest [17] with the age 65–84 population growing by 39 percent over the next 20 years and the over 85 population growing by 106 percent. Currently, 850,000 people in the UK are living with dementia and these numbers are predicted to rise to 2,060,903 in 2050 [18]. The rising numbers of the elderly, those with frailty and those with dementia, when associated with a population predicted to grow by 8 million over the next 20 years, a static birth rate of about 700,000 per year, and net immigration of 3.5 million over 20 years. As a result the working age population is expected to fall [19] this is the so-called demographic time bomb that is also an issue in other developed countries.
- Of more immediate impact on day-to-day clinical practice is the overall impact of these social forces and their impact on what I have called the "social revolution" of the twentieth century (see Chapter 2). Here we see cultural change, the retreat of the class divisions and the freeing up of the barriers to social mobility, the development of meritocracy, and the rise of the "grammar school" generation. Looking ahead to the cultural impacts that will underpin further evolution in the primary care sector we have to first reflect that such cultural adaptation is never quick and in some respects the sector's design and performance hark back to a different world where
  - Deference was more influential in the relationship between doctor and patient.
  - Professional status – doctor, nurse, pharmacist, dentist, etc. – carried authority, trust and respect.
  - Individual citizens queued for the bus or their turn to see the doctor were grateful for care and attention and obeyed "doctor's orders".
- Adapting to modern cultural trends will mean, over time
  - A new framework of *governance* in the sector – the framework of arrangements which ensure the sector is trustworthy and fit for purpose – more open to challenge and scrutiny, more responsive to the aspirations of

the community, more accountable for its use of resources and the quality of care it provides, safer by design, and reflecting the findings of the Cadbury Report into corporate governance [16].

* Responding to the "comprehensive school" generation – more egalitarian, more a partnership between service user and care provider, more respect for diversity and a more inclusive view of community.

TECHNOLOGICAL FACTORS

Just as it would be too simplistic to only consider the rise in the elderly population, the impact of austerity, and the Brexit agenda in earlier sections, so it would also be too narrow a perspective to only look at the impact of the *digital world* as the only technological force driving change in the sector. To some extent technological change is driven by economics and social forces, and to some extent technology drives political and economic change. These are not separate, independent factors affecting development, rather they are interdependent and complementary.

Before reflecting on the impact of the digital revolution on the sector now and in the foreseeable future there are other technologies to consider:

- New treatments – genetic healthcare, new drugs and new therapies such as regenerative medicine (for example for macular degeneration and osteoarthritis).
- Green technologies – a world where renewable energy, environmental impact assessments and sustainability are important aspects of healthcare, where our individual, personal impact and responsibility matter and where profligate use of scarce resources (e.g. oil, antibiotics and food) is discouraged by social pressure or taxation. It is interesting to consider how political and economic tools such as taxation have started to be used with significant impact on green and behavioural adaptation issues such as childhood obesity, plastic bag usage and diesel cars – integrated nudging.
- Similarly, we should not restrict our consideration of technologies to only structural ones. The knowledge economy – the learning or educational technology – is hugely influential by opening minds and expanding horizons, by marketing opportunity, and encouraging enquiry and fulfilment. The financial services sector is very significant in the British economy using finance and capital as a resource to reinforce investment and economic growth. Health technologies such as implantable treatments, wearable diagnostic aids and near-patient testing kits are all technologies which will have impact, often by liberating individuals from dependency on pills or professional clinicians.

Vignette

SB (aged fifty-four) called an out-of-hours GP service late on a Sunday evening with a severe urinary tract infection. She had lost one kidney to cancer a year ago and the other one had also been damaged. Her previous treatment had seen her move to the area and she did not carry any of her records, but she had been hugely reassured that a recent kidney scan was OK. Effective treatment options were significantly compromised by our knowledge vacuum. It is all very well having the technology, but we need it at the point of care where decisions about her care needed to be made late on a Sunday evening.

- However new digital technologies has, over recent years, had the greatest impact on society and the primary care sector. In our *inspection and analysis* of the sector it is this technology which is rewriting the ground rules, freeing individuals from having to rely on analogue, restricted opportunities which are only open when the gate is open. A world in the primary healthcare sector of gatekeeping and referral, of restricted access and boundaries between services, where health records are not shared. As was recently pointed out by the Commonwealth Fund in the United States [20], opening the health records market may have far-reaching consequences. The records have value, and moving control of them away from clinicians and providers towards the individual owner may disrupt the healthcare industry and liberate individuals from the yoke of professional capture [21].
- When the answer to any question is only a few mouse-clicks away, why wait to see your doctor to ask the question? When you can get your bank balance on your phone, why go to the branch? When you can buy your food online and have it delivered, why go shopping? In the modern world there has to be added value to justify shopping for the "experience" or visiting the bank to "get personal advice" or seeing your doctor for personal treatment.

This chapter has been about understanding the primary healthcare system, how it is currently responding to the situation it finds itself in and how fit it is for the challenges it is facing. The chapter ends the first part of the book. In the following chapter we shall look further at tools for deepening our understanding of the way the system is behaving, using the elements of system's thinking [5] (archetypes, paradigms, mental models, mindsets, leverage and personal mastery for example) so that in the final part of the book we can draw the threads together to offer a vision for the future of "home-based, liberated, deinstitutional" care.

REFERENCES

1. House of Commons Health Committee. 2016. Primary care: Fourth report of session 2015–16. HC 408. www.parliament.uk/healthcare.
2. Care Quality Commission. 2017. *The State of Care in General Practice 2014–2017*. CQC, London.
3. Hart JT. 1971. The inverse care law. *Lancet* 297:405–12. https://www.thelancet.com/journals/lancet/article/PIIS0140-6736(71)92410-X/fulltext.
4. Royal College Paediatrics and Child Health. 2014. *Intercollegiate guidance-Safeguarding Children and Young People: Roles and Competencies for Healthcare Staff*. 3rd ed. Royal College Paediatrics and Child Health, London.
5. Senge PM. 1990. *The Fifth Discipline*. Currency/Doubleday, New York.

6. OECD/European Observatory on Health Systems and Policies. 2017. *The State of Health in the EU; United Kingdom: Country Health Profile 2017.* OECD Publishing, Paris.
7. NHS England. 2014. *Five Year Forward View.* NHSE, London.
8. Care Quality Commission. 2018. *Local system reviews: Interim report.* CQC, London.
9. Care Quality Commission. 2018. *The state of care in independent online primary health services.* CQC, London.
10. Chartered Institute of Personnel and Development (CIPD). 2009. PESTLE analysis: History and application. www.cipd.co.uk/subjects/corpstrtgy/general/pestle-analysis.htm.
11. Kickbusch I. 2015. The political determinants of health – 10 years on. *BMJ*; 350.
12. Cream J, Maguire G and Robertson R. 2018. How have public attitudes to the NHS changed over the past three decades? https://www.kingsfund.org.uk/publications/how-have-public-attitudes-to-nhs-changed.
13. Rivett G. 1998. *From Cradle to Grave.* King's Fund, London.
14. Fletcher E, Abel GA, Anderson R et al. 2017. Quitting patient care and career break intentions among general practitioners in South West England: Findings of a census survey of general practitioners. *BMJ Open* 7:015853.
15. Bandolier, www.bandolier.org.uk.
16. Committee on the Financial Aspects of Corporate Governance. 1992. *The financial aspects of corporate governance.* Gee Professional Publishing, London.
17. King's Fund. 2018. Demography: Future trends. www.kingsfund.org.uk/projects/time-think-differently/trends-demography.
18. https://dementiastatistics.org.uk.
19. Office for National statistics, www.ons.gov.uk.
20. The Commonwealth Fund, www.commonwealthfund.org.
21. Illich I. 1976. *Limits to Medicine: Medical Nemesis.* Penguin, London.
22. NHS England. 2016. *General Practice Forward View.* NHSE, London.

5

Synergy

INTRODUCTION

If the beginning of the book has looked at the primary care sector from the perspective of its history and has offered an examination of its current status, this chapter sees a transition to considering the sector from a more physiological and dynamic, less anatomical or static standpoint. To initiate this transition I will start you on a journey that may take the rest of your life to complete – a journey into your mind, a journey to open up the way you think – to free you from the inevitable constraints that any life involves. Whether you are a clinician, a manager or other stakeholder in the British health and welfare system you will think about your world in ways which are determined by your own experience and along tracks which your training and experience has prepared you for. The transition does not require you to reject any of your past experiences or seek to devalue them in any way; it just asks you to be open to look at that experience from a different perspective using different lenses or tools. This is to prepare you for the following chapters where the tools of systems thinking will push your thinking further into using the analysis of the primary care sector to engage with the redesign or transformation proposed later in the book.

Before we delve into succeeding chapters to look at some tools for analysing the sector's performance as a system, in this chapter we look at some key thinking skills and then at a few examples where the *physiology, ecology* and *molecular biology* involved can add a scientific and clinical perspective to our analysis. While those from non-clinical backgrounds may find this chapter more challenging, I ask for your forgiveness. Just as clinicians have often used "clinical speak" as a cloak to hide behind and managers used "management speak", so we will be using these clinical and conceptual examples and disciplines to help clinicians and non-clinicians start the later chapters with an appreciation of their common interests. As before, in the text, I will illustrate with examples from my own experience to amuse you or stretch your thinking a bit.

While all physical objects react and respond to each other in response to the fundamental principles established and expounded by the writings and laws of Archimedes and Newton, biological systems are not rigid bodies and the way they behave is more analogous to complex adaptive systems [1] in that they comprise multiple elements interacting with each other and their environment in ways which are less linear – not just cause and effect but more dependent on their interactions and relationships.

CAUSE AND EFFECT

For many years scientists saw the universe as a linear place, one where simple rules of cause and effect apply. They viewed the universe as big machine and thought that if they took the machine apart and understood the parts, then they would understand the whole. They also thought that the universe's components could be viewed as machines, believing that if we worked on the parts of these machines and made each part work better, then the whole would work better. Scientists believed the universe and everything in it could be predicted and controlled.

Despite how hard they tried to find the missing components to complete the picture they failed. Despite using the most powerful computers in the world the weather remained unpredictable, despite intensive study and analysis, ecosystems and the immune systems did not behave as expected. But it was in the world of quantum physics that the strangest discoveries were being made and it was apparent that the very smallest subnuclear particles were behaving according to a very different set of rules to cause and effect. For example, we need to appreciate the following contributions:

- Greek thinkers such as Socrates, Plato and Aristotle who founded our approach to *critical thinking* – by questioning the status quo – challenging current thinking in a structured way to clarify areas and issues where conclusions may need to be reconsidered. This approach has underpinned much of the development of the world since their time. Science, art, theology and learning disciplines have all relied on criticism and critical thinking in order to evolve.

  Think of how you have learned and refined your approach as a result of reviewing a complaint or as a result of an audit or research project: As a young, inexperienced family doctor, a seminar led by an eminent moral philosopher [2] led to a critical review of my thinking about genetics. He probed and challenged me until I had to agree with him that it is our individual genetic inheritance received from our parents and passed on to our children that makes us unique.

- *Synergy*: The interaction or cooperation of two or more agents to produce a combined effect greater than the sum of their separate effects.

  Listen to a musical group where the instruments – including the voice – support and interact together to produce music where the musicians sublimate their solo excellence in support of the greater good. Or, consider that the greatest football striker can only be great in a great team, or that an "outstanding" Care Quality Commission (CQC) rating is often the result of synergy.

  A rural practice in Devon had managed to break the eighty percent barrier of people on its palliative care register who achieved their preferred place of death. The team – hospice and community nursing, GP, care coordinator, medicines manager, holistic therapist and volunteer facilitator – met each month to review the care plans for about twenty people. The team motto "make it happen" was driven by the needs of patients and their families. The team recognised their reliance on each other's contribution. Listening in to their discussions and talking to a few associated voluntary carers was one of my most humbling experiences.

- *Analogy*: A comparison between one thing and another especially for the purpose of explanation or clarification. From the Greek *analogous*, meaning "proportion" or "proportionate", having the same function but different evolutionary origins.

  The analogy between the report into corporate governance established in the wake of a series of corporate failures [3] and the description of clinical governance [4] bears reflection. While the former looked at the arrangements underpinning public confidence in corporate board performance (in the National Health Service [NHS] as much as in private business), so the latter looked at the arrangements assuring public confidence in clinical practice. Boards with responsibility for the latter had to necessarily be accountable for both. The analogy of the Cadbury Report can help clinicians understand that clinical governance is not just about individual performance or elements such as education or audit, rather it is about trustworthiness of the systems governing clinical practice just as corporate governance is about the trustworthiness of the board and management of the organisation.

- *Symmetry*: The correspondence in size, form and arrangement of parts on opposite sides of a plane, line or point; regularity of form or arrangement in terms of like, reciprocal or corresponding parts. Our bodies are largely symmetrical but not perfectly if you realise that you only have one heart, one of your feet is larger than the other and your fingerprints may differ, for example. Once you start to look at it, nature's beauty rests, at least in part, on its symmetry.

  When studying molecular biology I spent a pleasant few weeks surrounded by rolls of wallpaper analysing the patterns and planes of symmetry. Then I studied with Prof Lewis Wolpert [5] whose thinking spanned embryonic development, pattern formation and concepts of theoretical biology, together in a way which almost helped me understand him – why and how symmetry is a foundation for differentiation and early embryonic development.

- *Entropy*: This is a bit tricky, as we need to span thermodynamics, chemistry and biology alongside systems theory. While its origins are Greek – *entropia* "turning inwards" like an eyelid – it also encompasses disorder and the number of states a system can take on. Here, I think the best description is that the entropy of a system is the amount of energy consumed internally in running the system without producing any useful product. I find this a useful construct for analysing organisations and systems.

  Project in Leicester was trying to agree how to deliver elective care across a health economy. A hugely expensive group of stakeholders met monthly for a couple of years. Although the output was limited and hot air quotient entropy high, the impact was really impressive when a very small implementation team bottled the "hot air", drove plans through the local boards and took "executive" decisions. So we should not decry the energy consumed on building the internal energy of the organisation – it is a foundation for later impact.

- *Communication*: Communication is the exchange of information between transmitter and recipient. It all sounds so simple, but if you consider:
  - The serious case reviews into Baby P, Victoria Climbie or earlier examples like Maria Colwell or Rikki Neave where poor communications between the agencies responsible for protecting children are a common theme because of their ineffectiveness or absence. The lessons have never been learned, because the mechanisms, systems and features of the way the safeguarding systems are designed do not promote protection of the vulnerable.
  - The CQC reports into digital providers where communications between the private digital provider and the patient's NHS GPs are problematic at least in part because guidance from the GMC seeks to protect patient confidentiality rather than support joined-up, effective provision of care.
  - Communications between CQC and NHS England and local clinical commissioning groups (CCGs) when inadequate primary care provision is identified often resulted in blame, denial and anger, not a learning system, not effective communication. It was more a cathartic response to the years of neglect, which lie behind so many failing services.
  - The communication breakdowns which destroy marriages, professional partnerships and most relationships are the result of emotional dissonance [6]. It is too simplistic to talk of "give and take" or tolerance. Effective communication requires emotional maturity, trust and sublimation of individual self-interest for agreed mutual benefit.

We shall return to consider this communication issue further later in the book (Chapter 8) because the dynamics they describe are important to issues such as team working, integration between organisations and sectors and the importance of building strong partnerships.

COMPLEXITY THEORY

Gradually as scientists of all disciplines explored these phenomena (detailed above), a new theory emerged – complexity theory [1] – a theory based on relationships, emergence, patterns and iterations. It is a theory that maintains that the universe is full of systems (weather systems, immune systems, social systems, etc.) and that these systems are complex and constantly adapting to their environment. Hence, complex adaptive systems.

If we are to look at the primary care system (or the out-of-hospital care system or home-based care system) as an example of a complex adaptive system, then we need to appreciate its implications. We will start by looking at some relatively, but deceptively, simple biological systems to develop a common appreciation of the dynamics underpinning complex adaptive systems before we consider the design features they illustrate. We should then be able to pull together the concepts, issues and design features to help add depth to the analysis of the current primary care sector that Chapter 4 ended with.

HOMEOSTASIS

First, we need to understand how organisms maintain homeostasis, or a stable internal environment [7].

KEY POINTS

- *Homeostasis* is the tendency to resist change in order to maintain a stable, relatively constant internal environment.
- Homeostasis typically involves *negative feedback loops* that counteract changes of various properties from their target values, known as *set points* (resisting change).
- In contrast to negative feedback loops, *positive feedback loops* amplify their initiating stimuli. In other words, they move the system away from its starting state (reinforcing change).

Introduction

What's the temperature in the room where you're sitting right now? Probably not exactly 98.6°F or 37.0°C. Your body temperature is usually very close to these values. In fact, if your core body temperature doesn't stay within relatively narrow limits – from about 95°F (34°C) to 107°F (41.7°C) – the results can be dangerous or even deadly.

This tendency to maintain a stable, relatively constant internal environment is called *homeostasis*. The body maintains homeostasis for many factors in addition to temperature. For instance, the concentration of various chemicals in your blood must be kept steady, along with its acidity and the concentration of glucose, fats, waste products and oxygen. If these values rise too high or fall too low, you can end up getting very sick.

We need to appreciate that homeostasis is maintained at various levels, not just the level of the whole body as it is for temperature but within a particular organ, system or cell. For instance, the stomach maintains a pH that's different from that of surrounding organs, and each individual cell maintains ion concentrations different from those of the surrounding fluid. Maintaining homeostasis at each level is key to maintaining the body's overall function.

So, how is homeostasis maintained? Let's answer this question by looking at some examples.

Maintaining homeostasis

Biological systems like those of your body are constantly being pushed away from their balance points. For instance, when you exercise, your muscles increase heat production, nudging your body temperature upward. Similarly, when you drink a glass of fruit juice, your blood glucose goes up. Homeostasis depends on the ability of your body to detect and oppose these changes.

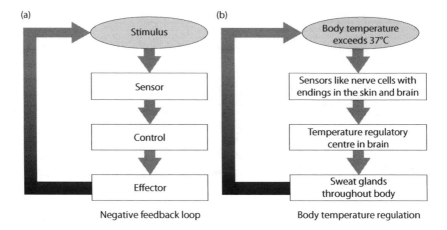

(a)   (b)

Negative feedback loop   Body temperature regulation

Figure 5.1 Homeostasis. **(a)** A negative feedback loop has four basic parts: a stimulus, sensor, control and effector. **(b)** Body temperature is regulated by negative feedback. The stimulus is when the body temperature exceeds 37°C, the sensors are the nerve cells with endings in the skin and brain, the control is the temperature regulatory centre in the brain, and the effector is the sweat glands throughout the body.

Maintenance of homeostasis usually involves *negative feedback loops* (Figure 5.1). These loops act to oppose the *stimulus*, or cue, that triggers them. For example, if your body temperature is too high, a negative feedback loop will act to bring it back down towards the *set point*, or target value, of 98.6°F or 37.0°C.

How does this work? First, high temperature will be detected by *sensors* – primarily nerve cells with endings in your skin and brain – and relayed to a temperature-regulatory *control centre* in your brain. The control centre will process the information and activate *effectors* – such as the sweat glands – whose job it is to oppose the stimulus by bringing body temperature down.

Of course, body temperature doesn't just swing above its target value; it can also drop below this value. In general, homeostatic circuits usually involve at least two negative feedback loops:

- One is activated when a parameter, like body temperature, is above the set point and is designed to bring it back down.
- One is activated when the parameter is below the set point and is designed to bring it back up.

To make this idea more concrete, let's take a closer look at the opposing feedback loops that control body temperature.

Homeostatic responses in temperature regulation

If you get either too hot or too cold, sensors in the periphery and the brain tell the temperature regulation centre of your brain, in a region called the hypothalamus, that your temperature has strayed from its set point.

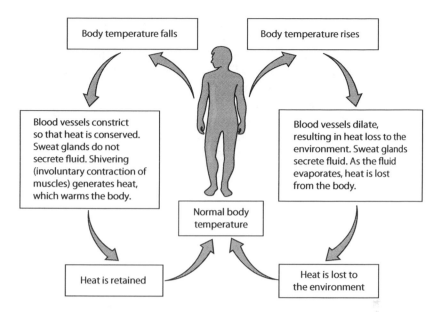

Figure 5.2 Temperature control.

For instance, if you've been exercising hard, your body temperature can rise above its set point, and you'll need to activate mechanisms that cool you down. Blood flow to your skin increases to speed up heat loss into your surroundings, and you might also start sweating, so the evaporation of sweat from your skin can help you cool off. Heavy breathing can also increase heat loss.

Figure 5.2 shows temperature regulation in response to signals from the nervous system. When the body temperature falls, the blood vessels constrict, sweat glands don't produce sweat, and shivering generates heat to warm the body. This causes heat to be retained and the body temperature to return to normal.

When the body temperature is too high, the blood vessels dilate, sweat glands secrete fluid and heat is lost from the body. As heat is lost to the environment, the body temperature returns to normal.

On the other hand, if you're sitting in a cold room and aren't dressed warmly, the temperature centre in the brain will need to trigger responses that help warm you up. The blood flow to your skin decreases, and you might start shivering so that your muscles generate more heat. You may also get goosebumps, that is when the hair on your body stands on end and traps a layer of air near your skin, and increases the release of hormones that act to increase heat production.

Your behaviour might also be affected. You might put on an extra sweater if you feel cold or change your diet to eat more salad in the heat for example.

Disruptions to feedback disrupt homeostasis

Homeostasis depends on negative feedback loops. So, anything that interferes with the feedback mechanisms can –and usually will! – disrupt homeostasis. In the case of the human body, this may lead to disease.

Diabetes, for example, is a disease caused by a broken feedback loop involving the hormone insulin (Figure 5.3). The broken feedback loop makes it difficult or impossible for the body to bring high blood sugar down to a normal level. To appreciate how diabetes occurs, let's take a quick look at the basics of blood sugar regulation. In a healthy person, blood sugar levels are controlled by two hormones: insulin and glucagon.

Insulin decreases the concentration of glucose in the blood. After you eat a meal, your blood glucose levels rise, triggering the secretion of insulin from β cells in your pancreas. Insulin acts as a signal that triggers cells of the body, such as fat and muscle cells, to take up glucose for use as fuel. Insulin also causes glucose to be converted into glycogen – a storage molecule – in the liver. Both processes pull sugar out of the blood, bringing blood sugar levels down, reducing insulin secretion and returning the whole system to homeostasis.

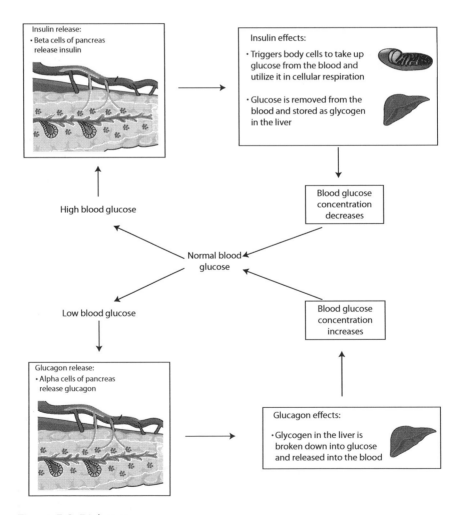

Figure 5.3 Diabetes.

If the blood glucose concentration rises above the normal range, insulin is released, which stimulates body cells to remove glucose from the blood. If blood glucose concentration drops below this range, glucagon is released, which stimulates body cells to release glucose into the blood.

Glucagon does the opposite: it increases the concentration of glucose in the blood. If you haven't eaten for a while, your blood glucose levels fall, triggering the release of glucagon from another group of pancreatic cells, the α cells. Glucagon acts on the liver, causing glycogen to be broken down into glucose and released into the bloodstream, causing blood sugar levels to go back up. This reduces glucagon secretion and brings the system back into balance.

Diabetes happens when a person's pancreas can't make enough insulin, or when cells in the body stop responding to insulin, or both. Under these conditions, body cells don't take up glucose readily, so blood sugar levels remain high for a long period of time after a meal. This is for two reasons:

- Muscle and fat cells don't get enough glucose, or fuel. This can make people feel tired and even cause muscle and fat tissues to waste away.
- High blood sugar causes symptoms like increased urination, thirst and even dehydration. Over time, it can lead to more serious complications.

Positive feedback loops

Homeostatic circuits usually involve negative feedback loops. The hallmark of a negative feedback loop is that it counteracts a change, bringing the value of a parameter – such as temperature or blood sugar – back towards normal.

Some biological systems, however, use positive feedback loops. Unlike negative feedback loops, *positive feedback loops* amplify the starting signal. Positive feedback loops are usually found in processes that need to be pushed to completion, not when the status quo needs to be maintained (Figure 5.4).

A positive feedback loop comes into play during childbirth. In childbirth, the baby's head presses on the cervix – the bottom of the uterus, through which the baby must emerge – and activates neurons to the brain. The neurons send a signal that leads to release of the hormone oxytocin from the pituitary gland.

Oxytocin increases uterine contractions, and thus pressure on the cervix. This causes the release of even more oxytocin and produces even stronger contractions. This positive feedback loop continues until the baby is born.

Normal childbirth is driven by a positive feedback loop. A positive feedback loop results in a change in the body's status, rather than a return to homeostasis. The feedback loop includes (the loop is drawn clockwise):

- Nerve impulses from the cervix being transmitted to the brain.
- The brain stimulates the pituitary gland to secrete oxytocin.
- Oxytocin is carried in the bloodstream to the uterus.
- Oxytocin stimulates uterine contractions and pushes the baby toward the cervix.
- The head of the baby pushes against the cervix.
- And so on in a loop!

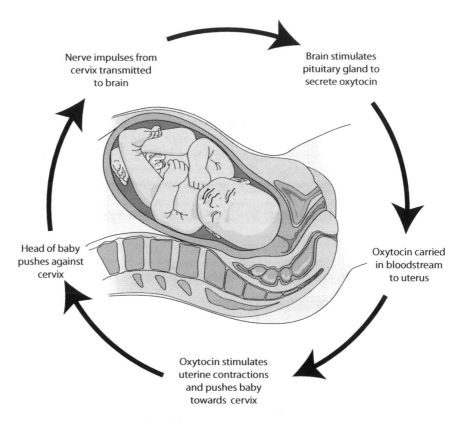

Figure 5.4 Positive feedback loops.

We now need to look at how a relatively simple biological system, responding homeostatically to its environment, becomes a complex adaptive system as it interrelates with other systems, what happens when things go wrong and how interventions have been designed to correct the problem. Let's next consider blood pressure.

HYPERTENSION

Blood is pumped round the body by the heart. The fluid (blood) flows through tubes (arteries, capillaries and veins) delivering oxygen and food to the cells of the body [8]. The size and elasticity of the blood vessels, the power of the pump and the rate at which it pumps determine the pressure in the system within a range which is normally maintained by negative feedback loops responding to environmental factors such as temperature and exercise. Blood vessels near the skin expand (vasodilate) in warm weather and constrict (vasoconstrict) in the cold to either increase heat loss or conserve heat.

However, other systems in the body can also affect blood pressure, for example adrenaline released at times of acute stress speeds up the heart and raises the blood pressure or a tumour releasing busts of adrenaline – a phaeochromocytoma – may be suspected when surges of high blood pressure are noted. On the other hand, in Addison's disease the lack of adrenocortical hormones can lead to acute episodes of shock with low blood pressure. In each situation the homeostatic mechanisms to maintain normal blood pressure are mediated by chemical messengers, that is, hormones and nerve impulses to dilate or constrict blood vessels. There are also additional kidney-mediated mechanisms which serve to regulate blood pressure by controlling the excretion of salt from the blood. Salt loss lowers blood pressure and salt retention raises it, and involve the renin/angiotensin system of powerful vasoconstricting chemicals which raise blood pressure and are inhibited by some of our most powerful antihypertensive drugs.

This is simply an example of how a comparatively simple "self-correcting" system, a homeostatic one with negative feedback loops, becomes a complex adaptive system as it relates to the other systems in the body. We could go further by considering ischaemic heart disease, cardiac failure and anaemia, but that is unnecessary here. It is enough to illustrate that at this level clinical speak is analogous to management speak: hypertension and its management is like any complex adaptive system (transport, finance, entertainment or politics) and we need to respect the transferability of insight that comes from experiencing and analysing a whole range of relevant disciplines.

A surgery practice uncovered a fraud issue and took immediate action to fix the problem. Then, out of the woodwork, came all the cultural and management issues behind the fraud. Two years later, following external analysis and support, interviews with all staff past and present, a cathartic redesign of the management of the practice and a new "vision", the staff survey at last became really positive. The archetype "fixes that fail" (see Chapter 7) illustrates the principle. It is similar to the tinkering with the Morris Minor model of the NHS which has gone on throughout the last seventy years – what is needed is a much more systematic and fundamental approach to not just resolve any issue but also ensure that it is "designed out" so that it cannot recur.

EVOLUTION

Volcanology, global warming, ecology and evolution dance to a different tune – homeostasis may fine-tune the bodies functioning minute by minute, just as modern electronics keep my car engine running efficiently, but in other spheres, adaptation, vital though it is to survival, is less immediate. Corporations, football clubs and political parties adapt to address their own pressures – to pay their dividend, to score in the game and win promotion/avoid relegation or to win the election, whereas in biology growth and cell division, maturation, ageing and sleep respond to the chemical tune of hormones and the ravages of pathology and external environmental pressures.

Over longer timescales, organisms adapt to their environment over the generations [9], the molecular biology of which we have now unravelled. DNA strands – beautifully elegant, balanced, symmetrical structures [10] – cascade down through the generations linking us to our ancestors but with mutation-mediated changes, genetic material exchange through crossover or chiasma, gene and DNA strand rearrangement, all driving evolutionary adaptation when meiotic production of germ cells (eggs and sperm) presages the next generation.

While Darwin's *On the Origin Species* [9] is sometimes paraphrased as "survival of the fittest" and describes the Galapagos Islands species divergence as a result of genetic (and physical) isolation, his rival Lamarck espoused adaptation and evolution by non-genetic means. Molecular biology has blurred the edges between these nineteenth century giants of biology, as epigenetics and mitochondrial inheritance have shown that classical Darwinian and Mendelian genetics cannot answer everything.

Nevertheless our understanding of the system of evolution is founded on the work of Darwin and Mendel, and is an example of a *complex adaptive system* where over time species adapt to the changing world they inhabit and develop new characteristics which increase their chance of survival.

The analogy to the evolution of the NHS and in particular to the home-based, primary care sector bears reflection. As time and generations pass, so the system needs to learn and adapt so that it remains fit for purpose as the world around it changes. We are not talking about the stable world of homeostasis or the relegation and promotion pressures of football or even the five-yearly electoral focus of politics. We are talking about the need to ensure that modern health and welfare systems reflect the needs of the community.

GENETIC HEALTHCARE

The opportunities for advances in molecular biology to transform clinical practice from the era of broad-spectrum antibiotics for infection and toxic chemotherapy for cancer into a world of therapy designed for individual treatment are now widely recognised. Inevitably the implementation phase of developments in genetic healthcare will be at a pace which satisfies regulatory and cultural requirements, but there will be a need for clinicians to learn and adapt during this phase.

It took a decade or more for clot busters, used at the time of a heart attack, to improve mortality and morbidity despite the evidence that they worked. It took at least as long for stroke prevention treatment to become accepted practice in people with non-rheumatic atrial fibrillation, again despite the evidence of safety and benefit. In other words, professional inertia and negative feedback loops, that is, homeostatic mechanisms, can delay the implementation of effective treatment. With the implementation of personalised genetic healthcare there will inevitably be similar hurdles in the way.

So, in summary, the mechanisms controlling the way biological and non-biological systems work comprise a range of approaches to maintaining the status quo and of adapting to changing circumstances, both in short periods of time and over long or very long periods of time. As we will see in later chapters, there are recurring themes and design features which can help us interpret and understand the issues involved. We also need to appreciate that some of the ground rules which we have all absorbed as part of our own lives are simply constructs to make sense of the circumstances we find ourselves in. We may not have tools in our bag to deal with rapid fundamental changes, such as the technological and social developments of the last seventy years. If we rely on evolution over generations to adapt to the digital post-family world then our out-of-hospital, home-based, primary care system will be as dead as the dodo.

ORGANISATIONAL FORM

The American architect Louis Sullivan is credited with the maxim that *form follows function* which became a mantra for many architects. But as Frank Lloyd Wright, the architect for the Guggenheim Museum [11], pointed out, form and function should be one, joined in a spiritual union. In the NHS primary care sector organisational forms have evolved over the last seventy years to fulfil the functions necessary to meet the welfare needs of the local community while they are living in that community. As members of the community have looked for more support from the sector, and as advances in clinical practice have allowed more care to be provided, so the capacity and capability of the sector has expanded. The question we need to consider is whether the *form and function* of the sector remain in a spiritual union. From the start of the NHS, care within the sector has been provided by a cocktail of NHS community staff, small businesses owned and providing services through contracts with the NHS, local authority employed staff, local voluntary sector organisations and their staff alongside individual and family members whose contribution is the vital glue holding the sector together.

The relationships between the staff providing services in the sector have either been through informal shared care arrangements or employer–employee line management systems, and the relationship between members of the community and the sector has been through:

- *Registration (with your GP practice or dentist)* – A continuing relationship with rights and responsibilities on both sides, an ongoing record of care and an employed team of clinicians and staff.
- *Referral (from your social worker or community nurse)* – Providing care usually for a defined period of time to an agreed plan determined by the referral process.
- *Informal choice (for example with your chemist shop)* – You are free to attend whichever you prefer.

Staff in the sector sometimes meet up socially across organisational boundaries, but meetings to agree on care plans and coordinate provision are unusual. The primary healthcare team of the 1970s, 1980s and early 1990s was never as much of a team as an orchestra, more a loose alliance like faith leaders grouping on remembrance Sunday. But memory makes the heart grow fonder and the current team working seems to be weak by design. For example, the CQC inspection found that the practice nurses hardly ever met with the GPs, or each other. The practice managers did their annual appraisal and they liaised with the care team through EMIS Web notes and emails. The GPs communicated with community nurses, midwives, health visitors and social workers by phone or fax; they did not use the same IT system and never met as a care team. When a diabetic mother had a stillbirth and the rest of her children had to be referred to the safeguarding team because of the risks involved consequent on domestic abuse, the GP realised she was one of eleven clinicians involved with the care of the family – and had never met most of them until the crisis brought them together.

Developing Cultures of High-Quality Care (2013) [12] and *Caring to Change* (2017) [13] and similar research into culture leadership have important resonances for any team working in the NHS. But there are also important lessons for the *pseudo teams* operating in the sector where team working is not driven by design; where objectives are not aligned across organisational boundaries; and where budgets, cultures and performance management approaches are too often in conflict rather than spiritual union.

If the dominant player in the sector has been general medical practice and its predominant organisational form is the *professional partnership*, then we might look to the evidence that such organisations are responding to the challenge, that the NHS was investing in their capacity and capability to respond, and that the opportunity to have real impact on the welfare of the community was motivating and proving attractive to clinicians, but the evidence is lacking.

- The popularity of general practice partnership as a career option is in decline [14], and while the predictions of some [15] that the model of GP partnership will disappear within ten years may be premature, the findings of the CQC inspection programme (see previous chapters) illustrate the stresses driving evolution.

- The drivers – rising numbers of frail elderly people with complex health and welfare needs, the shortening length of stay in hospital and the impact of technology enabling a greater range of care being provided in the community – are all expanding the responsibilities involved in providing care in the sector but without the powers necessary to deliver.

- Partnership working (partnership was discussed in Chapter 3 from a historical perspective, here we are looking at its fitness for the future), be it in personal or professional relationships, is founded on agreement between the parties to advance their common interests by trusting each other enough to share responsibility. It is a commitment which requires investment, a legal framework to underpin its validity and it is expensive to dissolve. If clinicians are uncertain about their future, worried about the risks involved in joining a partnership or wary of long-term commitment, then life as an employee may be more attractive. Because partners share the profits of the business, they also suffer when profits are falling. In the last decade the government's austerity agenda has meant falling profits in the sector, as costs increase at a time of flatline funding growth. My own small survey among fifty GP partners has shown an average twenty percent fall in take-home pay over the last decade, while non-partners have seen a fifteen percent increase in pay during this time. (also see Watson [16] for a recent review of the partnership model, which takes a detailed, if rather restricted and biased, view of the role of partnership in professional practice).

- However, when considering the balance sheet of professional partnership as an organisational form, we need to take a balanced view: the weaknesses of lack of accountability, weak staff and patient empowerment, a lack of openness to scrutiny and a culture of isolation from the rest of the sector and wider health economy; and the strengths of independence from NHS management frameworks, long-term relationships, commitment and trust forming the basis for strong relationships.

Similar considerations apply to other professional partnerships in the sector. Increasingly community pharmacy businesses and opticians are consolidating into multiple chains as result of market forces, and the rise of digital providers will reinforce the move towards professional "medicines managers" and "eye care clinicians" as opposed to dispensing pharmacists and opticians. Dentistry is also moving away from professional partnership towards the economies of scale of the corporate providers and chains.

Clinicians working in the community who are employed by NHS trusts, the hospice movement or social services are managed by their employers. Their objectives and priorities are agreed as part of their performance management arrangements, and the culture and leadership of their organisations is the major determinant, not just of their morale and approach to their work but also of their commitment to other clinicians they work alongside in the community. Good working relationships, a history of collaborative care, shared care plans and patient records are all seen and recognised as beneficial. But if they are not supported by management, then they are like poppies in a meadow – supported by the grass rather than the farmer.

Similarly, the design of the sector does not encourage mature relationships between local people and care providers – people become patients with all the dependency and "sickness mode" associations that entails. Adult behaviour, such as taking responsibility for your own health, medication, dialysis, near-patient testing for anticoagulation or glucose monitoring lags behind accepted behaviour in other countries, while demand for care is inflamed by the need for certification and a diagnostic label for legitimacy. Sticking plaster solutions to the rising tide of demand include walk-in centres, NHS 111, GP out-of-hours centres and paramedic home visiting as an outreach from ambulance trusts – all of them well-meaning but playing on the same football field with different coloured balls.

CONCLUSION

The extent to which the sector is fit for purpose has to be questioned. If the design of the sector is to reflect architecture where *form follows function* or if it should be one *joined in spiritual union*, then lessons from biology, organisational psychology, business and football need to be learned. Symmetry to improve efficiency, entropy to reduce waste, analogy and the study of complex adaptive systems to aid learning all matter alongside homeostasis evolution and genetic healthcare. If the sector is to once again become as fit for purpose as it was when it began, then our analysis, refined by the use of the tools described in the next three chapters has to become the design to deliver the vision of the final chapters.

REFERENCES

1. The Health Foundation. 2010. Complex adaptive systems. www.health.org. uk/sites/default/files/ComplexAdaptiveSystems.pdf.
2. Dunstan GR. 1985. Evolution and mutation in medical ethics. In S Doxiadis (ed), *Ethical Issues in Preventive Medicine*. Springer, Netherlands, pp. 11–18.
3. Committee on the Financial Aspects of Corporate Governance. 1992. *The financial aspects of corporate governance [Cadbury Report]*. Gee Professional Publishing, London.
4. Scally G and Donaldson L. 1998. Clinical governance and the drive for quality improvement in the new NHS in England. *BMJ* 317(7150):61–65.
5. Wolpert L. 1969. Positional information and spatial pattern of cellular differentiation. *J Theoretical Biology* 25(1):1–47.
6. The Relationship Foundation, www.relationshipfoundation.org.
7. Homeostasis. 2019. www.khanacademy.org.
8. Harvey W. 1973. *The Circulation of the Blood and Other Writings 1628*. Littlehampton books.
9. Darwin C. 1869. *On the Origin of the Species*. 1859 Folio society.
10. Watson JD and Crick FHC. 1953. A structure for deoxyribose nucleic acid. *Nature* 171(3): 737–8.
11. Wright FL. 1958, July 15. Frank Lloyd Wright to Harry Guggenheim. In *Frank Lloyd Wright: From within Outward* [exhibition catalog], 2009, Solomon R. Guggenheim Foundation, New York, p. 268.
12. West M. 2013. *Developing Cultures of High-Quality Care*. King's Fund, London. https://www.kingsfund.org.uk/blog/20/3/`3/developing-cultures-high quality-care-what do-leaders-have-to-do-to.
13. West M. 2017. *Caring to Change*. King's Fund, London.
14. Fletcher E, Abel GA, Anderson R et al. 2017. Quitting patient care and career break intentions among general practitioners in South West England: Findings of a census survey of general practitioners. *BMJ Open* 7:015853.
15. Roberts N. 2013. Dr Mike Bewick: GPs must act now to shape their future. *GP Online*, November 8.
16. Watson N. 2019. GP Partnership. www.gov.uk/dhsc.

6

Learning to support
effective care

INTRODUCTION

Too many of us stop learning too early in our lives either because of social circumstances or because we join a career path which does not require or encourage it. People who continue to study and learn longer benefit greatly from it, their employer benefits and so, in the case of doctors, do their patients, service users or customers. Learners gain insight, perspective and have their minds opened to new concepts and ideas. Just as apprentices in many trades move on to master their craft – be it in engineering or thatching, brewing or surgery – a master's qualification requires students to undertake independent reading and study, to be able to interpret qualitative and quantitative research, to reflect and interpret their disciplines and knowledge base, and undertake a project based on original thinking in their discipline. This is a foundation for the master to continue to learn throughout their life using the tools that studying at a master's level has given them. Within the primary care sector it has been most unusual for anyone to continue to study at this level and continue to learn throughout their life. Some GP trainers may be an exception as some areas require at least a diploma in medical education to become a trainer, and some managers do MBAs. But the vast majority of practitioners restrict their ongoing study and learning, post-appointment to substantive posts, to support the requirements of their position for annual appraisal, revalidation and for personal development in areas which interest them. On Care Quality Commission (CQC) inspection it has been a chastening experience to meet and interview so many committed, experienced professionals who have never been encouraged or eligible for extended studying opportunities. In the early 1990s, I suggested that GPs, like hospital consultants, might have access to a programme of leadership training as part of the GP fundholding scheme [1], but this was never taken up, and we still do not have a cadre of experienced, trained leaders in the sector able to stand comparison to the medical directors of acute trusts and their teams of clinical leaders.

In this chapter we shall briefly explore aspects of the whole *out-of-hospital* sector which determine its fitness for operating as a *learning system*, a system which is continually expanding its capacity to create its own future, not merely to survive through adapting to circumstance (i.e. *adaptive* learning) but through learning which enhances the system's capacity to create (i.e. *generative* learning) [2] or to move beyond the present context and situation to transform the design of the world the system lives in (i.e. *transformative* learning). Inevitably the exploration will be brief and limited, but is offered because it is important that the elements are considered together before we move onto the design features required in the transformed system in succeeding chapters. Because the sector is made up of a range of individuals from many different disciplines working together in loose teams – or pseudo teams [7] – we will start by looking at individual or personal mastery before moving on to aspects of team working and a few of the consequences, to relationships in the sector.

PERSONAL MASTERY

Just as becoming a master thatcher comes by continual practice, so personal mastery requires us to practice a set of disciplines which lay the foundations for continually expanding our mastery of ourselves. This begins by understanding ourselves and describing our vision – not our objectives or goals but more about our purpose or our direction. They are not the same but are both important: vision is a specific destination, a picture of where we want to be, whereas purpose is more abstract, such as excellence or improving health. Vision is multifaceted; material aspects like housing, income, possessions and ownership are complemented by personal factors like health, freedom, relationships, personal confidence and respect, and then there are contributions such as helping others in the community or contributing as a member of a profession or society. Describing one's own personal vision and using it to help build a coherent group vision, owned and refined by those we live and work with is a key aspect of personal mastery. But such group, team or organisational visions are never perfectly aligned to our own personal visions and this can cause difficulties. The discipline of personal mastery is, of course, much more than just establishing and our maintaining personal vision [2]; it is an essential first step, and its weakness or relative absence in the primary care sector is important given the lessons from CQC (see Chapter 4) and the pressures the sector is currently experiencing. Senge [2] also describes nine other elements making up the discipline – from commitment to the truth to fostering personal mastery in an organisation – but in the current situation and the future *digital world* we are considering it is all the individual *visions* and the personal disciplines of understanding ourselves, our personalities and our motivations, our attitudes and our aspirations which fuel our journey towards personal mastery.

PERSONAL MASTERY – THE ELEMENTS [2]
• Personal vision
• Holding creative tension
• Structural conflict
• Commitment to the truth
• Using the subconscious
• Integrating reason and intuition
• Seeing our connectedness to the world
• Compassion
• Commitment to the whole
• Fostering personal mastery in an organisation

TEAMS

Personal mastery will never be sufficient. In the provision of health and social care it is teams which deliver care – teams made up of individuals who add value by working together and gaining synergy from other team members' input. Working in teams is essential for the provision of safe, effective and person-centred care Individual citizen health problems challenge all our individual efforts, and when complex co-morbidities are involved we all need team expertise. Teams are complex and you may be confident contributing in some ways but more diffident in others. You may want to start by focusing on areas you feel you need to develop, for example, you may feel confident working in a team with your immediate work colleagues, but not in working with teams with other disciplines or agencies. Team working activities covering a wide range of issues that you will encounter in practice and that you will find easier to deal with if you have thought about them beforehand – so your own personal mastery is important to enable you to bring your expertise and experience to bear in a way which delivers added value or synergy.

Throughout the CQC inspection programme in English general practice we have heard of examples of effective team working both within the practice and with staff from other agencies. This has been particularly strong when it results from a focus on particular problem areas such as cancer care or in response to previous national programmes such as national service frameworks for diabetes, or for particular special groups or circumstances like university students or people with learning difficulties. The lack of focus on some key national priorities has meant examples of strong team working in those areas is lacking. Obesity, dementia, drug dependency, alcohol abuse and adolescent mental health issues would be examples where a more coordinated approach to team working across the sector and organisational boundaries is worthy of consideration. This not to underplay the significant work done by many practices in each of these areas, but more needs to be done. Many practices have expressed regret to CQC about the difficulties they are experiencing in promoting team working with partner providers. Health visiting, midwifery, community nursing, social worker and mental health practitioners would be examples where team working has become more difficult in recent years. Tools such as personality profiling [3] and preferred team roles [4] can be helpful in supporting individuals and teams to enhance their effectiveness in team situations. But until a framework is put together to support teams in delivering better outcomes and until a coherent framework of managing teams as teams across professional organisational and employment boundaries is put in place, these tools risk being seen as irrelevant.

While really strong examples of children's centre provision have been found, such as tackling issues of disadvantage and neglect, their links with general practice and primary care teams are too often weaker than they used to be. The CQC has heard of examples where previously health visitors were based in practices, met GPs frequently and ran joint baby clinics with them, and there was close liaison about any safeguarding or child development concerns. In recent times we hear that joint working and shared care of cases are more difficult. This is of particular concern given the importance of child protection and the repeated recommendations from serious case reviews [5] about the need for coordinated care and better communications between the various professionals and agencies involved.

Effective team working with community nurses seems much more common. Their focus on personal care for the frail elderly/housebound requires sharing of care on a regular basis with GPs and practice nurses, and CQC inspections have found most practices have effective systems to support communication, planning and support. Many of the most vulnerable people require both medical and social support if they are to lead fulfilling lives, but effective links between social workers, social care providers and primary care teams seem exceptional rather than routine. Although care planning among the members of the practice team seems common for the vulnerable frail elderly, it is too often described as being unrelated to their social care provision.

Similarly, other groups whose health needs span the remit of different primary care providers – for specialist mental health issues or substance misuse problems or eating disorders or dementia, for example, too often fail to get "best care" because of weak team working between organisations sharing responsibility. While CQC has seen widespread good practice supporting palliative care with specialist input from medical, nursing and social care providers, such practice seems notably lacking in other situations [6].

SHARED CARE

Shared care is a common situation in most areas I have visited. The charity Addaction provided support for patients with substance misuse problems in my local area, but it struggled to engage with local GP practices to "share care" with them. Most of the practices refused to prescribe methadone and several of the patients involved had been on a roundabout of exclusion from being registered at any one practice and having to be continually reallocated to another practice every few months for many years. Training [7] programmes to help practitioners become more proficient and confident in caring for this group of patients and support from the local primary care trust (PCT) helped challenge the prevailing mindset, which was acknowledged to be negative and damaging by and for everyone involved. As a result, the Addaction support workers started working with all the local practices in support of individuals who needed and benefited from this shared care approach.

The transition from isolated individual care through shared care to team working requires a shared approach to care planning and decision making and the fostering of a culture of mutual support for those involved in implementing action plans. Moving along this path requires the following.

Alignment

Teams that are relatively unaligned don't share common culture and thinking; lack a common set of values and priorities; or suffer from conflicts of interest that prevent coherence, waste energy and become ineffective. By contrast, when teams become more aligned a commonality of direction emerges and individual energies are more harmonised, and so a resonance or synergy develops. The team's output is thus more coherent, like the light of a laser compared to a candle. There emerges a shared vision as an extension of individuals' visions. Indeed empowerment of individuals in teams requires a sufficient degree of alignment to produce commitment to each team member and to their shared vision. If an orchestra or band is to gel, then the members need to be aligned and committed. Within any aligned team in the primary care sector dealing with the complex issues involved in providing care, there will be a requirement to analyse and critically review care needs and care plans. This process of analysis and critical thinking will help develop team identity.

The following story is an example of alignment: The school nurses from the large local comprehensive school approached the local GP practice with concerns about teenage mental health issues. Too many teens were diagnosed with anxiety and depression, had eating disorders or were self-harming. Over a year or two, a group of 200 young people were helped to deal with their problems though a team-based approach to care which included psychoanalytical counselling, behavioural therapy, cognitive behavioural therapy, art and music therapy, exercise programmes, nutrition and dietetic sessions, individual and group therapy sessions and family therapy as well as medication. The team liaised with specialist colleagues from health and education, and over time was able to demonstrate impressive results, both in terms of reducing referrals to Child and Adolescent Mental Health Services (CAMHS) and in helping young people during their transition from school to further education or work.

Discussion

Discussion involves talking together, while *dialogue* means learning together. They are two essential processes through which teams can translate decisions into actions. They are both essential for effective team working. Discussion has the same derivation as percussion or concussion. It suggests a free flow of conversation during which issues may be analysed and dissected from the many different perspectives contributed by all those who take part. The purpose of the discussion is often to come to a decision followed by one or a series of actions. A sustained emphasis on "winning" is not compatible with giving enough priority to alignment and coherence, and too much dominance by any individual will need development to be challenged and modified by the team.

Dialogue

Bohm [8], a physicist, suggests that what is needed to bring about a change of priorities is dialogue, which is different from discussion. Dialogue is derived from the Greek *dialogos*: *dia* meaning "through" and *logos* meaning "word". In dialogue, Bohm contends, a group accesses a larger "pool of common meaning" which cannot be accessed individually. The purpose of dialogue is to go beyond any one individual's understanding; it is a group activity where we are seeking synthesis of individual's ideas to gain greater insight. We are looking for a common meaning where members of the group or team are no longer primarily in opposition nor can they be said to be simply interacting, rather they are participating in creating a pool of common meaning. Through dialogue a group can explore complex, difficult issues from many different points of view. Individuals suspend their assumptions and preconceived ideas to communicate more freely. The result is a free exploration which can bring to the surface the full depth of people's experience and thought and yet can move beyond their individual views.

Bohm identifies three basic considerations that are essential for dialogue to flourish:

1. Participants must suspend their own assumptions and open themselves to become receptive to the exchange of ideas involved in the dialogue.
2. All participants must regard themselves as colleagues – hierarchies and power blocks can inhibit dialogue. Colleagues have to respect each other's professionalism and experience, and value each other as team members if they are to learn from each other through dialogue.
3. Someone has to "hold the context" of the dialogue. This can be an external facilitator, but experienced teams can hold this role within the team. This role is essential to help keep the team dialogue on track, and to avoid defensive or comfort-seeking patterns of behaviour.

If primary care teams are to learn together, they will need to balance dialogue and discussion, and develop a group or team identity as a result. Dialogue helps to develop trust that carries over into discussions and supports better decision making, more productive actions are planned, and better care will be provided. Sadly, membership in such a team is a risky business for individuals, particularly if they are insecure in their own identity and unsure of their own personal viewpoints. We all tend to retreat to defensive behaviour when challenged and this can prevent the kind of *team learning* which is required if teams are to move beyond symptomatic solutions to the problems they face, for example, who will visit whom and what will they do on to more systematic analysis and solutions such as empowerment and partnership.

Practise makes perfect

It cannot be stressed too much that team learning is a team skill. A group of talented individual learners will not necessarily produce a learning team any more than a group of talented athletes will produce a great team. Learning teams have to learn how to perform together – an orchestra cannot just perform, it has to practise, as does a great football team.

In the primary care sector, teams may have worked together for a long time and will have to break out from their historic ways of working together if they are to become more effective.

Donald Schon [9] described the essential principles of practice as experimentation in a virtual world. Primary healthcare teams could do worse than discuss some of the vignettes and examples scattered through this book as examples of virtual situations they could learn from by practice. They might find they develop a deeper understanding of each other and begin to experience some "team learning". For example, using the two scenarios "Choice first" and "The feel good factor" [10] may also be a useful way of thinking through the choices involved in determining our own future as an aid to building your own shared vision.

Mental models and mindsets

While mental models are one of the five disciplines underpinning systems thinking [2], "the art & practice of the learning organisation" are essentially our own personal toolkit through which we make decisions, built up from our learning and experience and to some extent trapped and fixed by that, mindsets are the amalgam of the attitudes we hold. Mindsets have been described as either fixed or generative but in reality need to be developmental if we are to adapt to change in the environment we live in. Using the range of mental models and mindsets represented in the teams we work with during our career to support the building of a shared vision of our purpose is the essential "transformation" which we need to undertake if we are to build effective teams able to move from pseudo teams to real teams [6], teams which behave like an orchestra rather than a collection of musicians or a champion football team rather than a relegation candidate.

If a general practice believes that patients are partners in delivering healthcare, they are likely to act differently from a practice that believes it is the provider of healthcare and patients are the recipients. If a practice feels it is in the business of promoting healthy lives, then it will act differently from one that believes it is in the business of caring for people with disease. If a pharmacy believes that it is in the business of boosting shareholders' value, then it will act differently from a pharmacy that believes it is there to manage medicines effectively. If a nursing team believes it is there to promote individual autonomy and the happiness of patients referred to it, then it will act differently from a team that views its task as providing personal care and comfort for those same patients. Of course, the choice is never binary – these are not either/or situations and the approach, choices and decisions we make as individuals, teams, organisations and networks are never as black or white as this implies. But this does not mean that our collective mental models and our combined collection of attitudes (our mindsets) can be ignored – they matter to how we perform now and particularly how we adapt to change. In the digital world where so many of the things we have relied on through our lives are changing – from High Street shops to how we bank or communicate, from how we access information to how we make choices. Problems arise because the mental models and mindsets involved are static or tacit, and they are not questioned, challenged or subjected to critical review or analysis. They are stuck, and do not respond and change as the environment changes. Because these perceptions remain tacit, unchanged as the world around them changes, and while they may have been appropriate in the past, they may now be inappropriate, damaging, harmful or past their sell-by date. So, while the patronising paternalism of Dr Finlay may have been appropriate in rural Scotland at the start of the NHS, it may no longer be an appropriate design for modern general medical practice in the digital, "post nuclear family" society we now have. While nursing owes some of its perspectives to its origins through the Poor Laws and Florence Nightingale with the virtues of charitable giving and voluntary effort, and while health visiting has enjoyed the perspective of social education and advice in the support of social change, such heritage and perspectives need to be challenged in the consumerist, post-industrial, digital society we now live in. Mental models and mindsets become part of the culture of the team and organisation, but they have to evolve, adapt, and change as circumstances do, otherwise they do not remain fit for purpose.

Failure to appreciate the importance of the variety of perspectives involved and the necessity of challenging and analysing them has been a problem in the primary care sector over the years, and this has made team working and coordination of care across the sector problematic. Trying to develop a systematic approach to care within the sector is always going to be difficult when individuals, groups and organisations within the sector have very different mindsets, mental models and perceptions about their roles and responsibilities in the area under consideration.

Individual, group and team mental models and mindsets are often deeply held, cherished and central to their identity and so can be resistant to change to an extent which sometimes defies reason: For example, there has been a recruitment problem in general practice recent years. While this has affected many disciplines in the sector – from practice managers to health visitors and practice nurses – it has been the difficulty of recruiting general practitioners and particularly GP partners which has been grabbing headlines. "We need more resources" has been the scream from GPs, local medical committees and their national representatives. As the CQC inspection programme has found and as illustrated by the decline in popularity of the sector among the public in the British Social Attitudes survey [11] and as recommended by the House of Commons inquiry into the sector [12], extra resources cannot be the complete answer. Although additional resources may well be part of the solution – and the scale of four percent above inflation is widely thought to be the ballpark requirement – reform through challenging attitudes and behaviours and analysis of the mental models involved and the governance arrangements underpinning practice is also required if the recruitment problems are to be overcome so as to ensure a sustainable workforce. This kind of approach to redefining professionalism is what it means to be a general practitioner is fundamental to this analysis and a challenge which forms part of the vision for the sector's future sketched out in Chapter 10. The thinking behind this illustrates the distinction between adaptive, generative and transformative thinking. While the strident call for more resources is an understandable reaction to "how it feels" to be working in a stretched sector facing ever-rising demand with shrinking resources (this is an adaptive response), the generative response recognises the scope for efficiency improvements through improved ways of working and integration. But true transformative thinking requires acceptance that evolution and step-by-step change is not enough. What is required is the transformation of the sector, a redesign to be fit for the future, a Tesla rather than a Mark 30 Morris Minor held together by sticking plaster. This moves thinking beyond evolutionary adaptive, incremental change to a more transformative approach – a knight's move or in genetic terms "translocation" rather than point mutation.

Systems thinking

Before we move into the realm of the practice of systems thinking in the sector, by looking at archetypes and paradigms in the next chapter, we need to bring together some of the aforementioned elements. First, we need to recognise that some of the tools and approaches we are considering are essentially personal activities, others require groups or team participation. Team learning and building shared vision for example require a merging and learning framework, which requires all participants to adopt new ways of thinking, new rules of engagement and to refresh the values and assumptions that have hitherto guided their behaviour and decision making. We also have to acknowledge the issue of pace. We do not all learn in the same way or at the same pace, and the vision we are building takes time to emerge – like an elephant, it can only be eaten one bite at a time.

While walking the South West Coast Path last year I was talking to members of a walking group about their vision of the role of the National Health Service in our digital future. Doug was sure that disease management and personal safety would remain key concerns in his old age, while Sophie emphasised the importance of trustworthiness and relationships, both personal and between organisations. Annie helped the group realise that in our digital future we would remain at risk from system failures (how percipient given the recent TSB Bank and Facebook examples of IT dysfunction) unless we, as individual people, remained in control. All the group members came together by the end of the day, but everyone's journey had been different. The group's convenor, Arthur, a retired physicist and engineer put it like this: "We have all led very different lives and written and lived our own biographies, so all our visions are going to differ in some respects. But I know we are all hoping for a service which respects its heritage and learns from it – adapts to the modern, digital world and is fit for the future whatever it may bring".

So systems thinking is about seeing the whole picture as well as the detail (the wood and the trees) and realising that each element is dependent on the others – nothing in the vision is independent. We are all part of this sector, all involved in its future, and all involved in designing and creating it. The key message is that it is *our* future that we are considering, our system that is evolving, and we must all be part of the dialogue through which the shared vision is built, the learning takes place and our learning organisation evolves.

Personal responsibility

Alfred Mele [13] argues cogently for the gap between self-control and the autonomous agent being only partially bridged by the concept of personal autonomy. But certainly in our everyday life, the concept of us each being individually responsible for our own actions and behaviours is well accepted. In the primary care sector the idea that individuals have at least some responsibility for their own health is not new and indeed is a central feature of maturity – we accept parental responsibility until young people are mature enough to make their own decisions and assume responsibility for their own lives. Of course, there are limits. Some health problems are not our own fault, injuries and accidents happen, we catch infections sometimes through no fault of our own and develop cancers or other conditions as our life moves ahead without any personal culpability. Nevertheless we all accept that there are things we are responsible for and should take steps to adopt or avoid so that we maximise our potential. We do have responsibility for our own lifestyle – how we live our lives – and should recognise that avoiding harmful addictions, and maintaining a healthy diet, weight and level of physical fitness do matter, as does behaving in socially acceptable ways to others we relate to or have responsibility for. If we accept the concept of being responsible for those parts of our health and life that we can control, then assuming the same exceptions about maturity, it is surely right that our relationship with our health and welfare service should be one where our personal responsibility is respected, promoted and valued. Until now, the services have behaved somewhat arrogantly towards those who use them. These have not been relationships of equal partners – the doctor–patient, the pharmacist–customer and the optician–client relationships for example each imply that the clinician has the responsibility and power in the relationship. In the emerging digital world, the power that we each enjoy – to choose our entertainment or news channel, to select our own shopping online and to gamble "responsibly" – comes with new responsibilities, for example to protect our passwords. In this digital world our concept of personal responsibility for our health and welfare needs to mature – to grow beyond the dependency of the doctor–patient relationship [15].

Immaturity and maturity

John G had had a problem with opiates for the last ten years. The addiction had destroyed many parts of his life – he had dropped out of education, employment and his family. He used all his money to fund his addiction and his personal relationships were all pretty immature. When working with John, I found him full of supressed anger and blame. He blamed everybody for his addiction, his destitution and his misery. He adopted the role of the victim, even to the extent that he found it impossible to keep appointments or pick up prescriptions. Over three years of weekly sessions – with the carrot of a script each time – John and I focussed on the positives: on aspects of maturity (personal hygiene), respecting other people and his own personal growth. After the three years, John was far from being a mature adult and far from leaving his old world behind, but at least he was more positive, accepted that blaming everyone else for his problems was wrong, and had stayed out of prison. Now, ten years later, John has a family, has stopped using, and indeed moved away from smoking and alcohol completely. He is working and helping a local youth project. When I met him recently he told me that he knew he had had a lot of growing up to do, but he was getting there and knew his future was his to build. While drug addiction may seem an extreme example of immature mindsets and mental models, we are all walking along the same road to maturity at our own pace, and just as we need to foster a learning culture (see earlier) so we need to recognise, incentivise and reward maturity [15].

Advocacy

Advocacy is another dimension to the emerging relationship between each individual in the community and the health and welfare service. There are many situations where advocacy may matter. An advocate is someone who provides advocacy support when you need it. An advocate might help you access information you need or go with you to meetings or an interview in a supportive role. You may want your advocate to write letters on your behalf or speak for you in situations where you don't feel able to speak for yourself. In the health and welfare service, the role of an advocate and the importance of advocacy have increased over recent years. While your GP has always had a role to be your advocate – to ensure you get access to services, to write letters on your behalf and perhaps to attend meetings – representing your interest, in the future digital world this will become an even more important role. While we may each file our own tax returns online, manage our own bank accounts and shopping, we may struggle to get to see the right health service. Do we need to see a surgeon or a physician? Do we need an optician or an ophthalmologist? Doe my elderly mother need a home package of care or a place in a care home? In the vision for the service briefly sketched out in Chapter 10, there is mention of the need for each of us to have someone who can act as our advocate. This may be our family doctor or we might choose a nurse, a social worker or another professional who can advise us and take action on our behalf; someone we trust and empower to make decisions for us. Many of us hold lasting power of attorney (LPA) for elderly relatives, either to cover finance or health and welfare or both. I certainly do for three family members. What this health and welfare advocacy role would mean extending this concept of LPA to all members of society to choose a welfare practitioner to act on our behalf, and of course the right to change that holder when we want to. While in NHS Mk 1 we have all had the right to register with a GP and his/her practice along with all that implies about responsibility and accountability, I am now suggesting that advocacy – support for us, with us and through a relationship with us – will become a key feature of our more adult relationship with the sector in future. This does mean that we would have to give some element of control to our advocate, but ultimate responsibility will be our own to a much greater extent than in NHS Mk 1.

Empowerment

The term *empowerment* refers to measures designed to increase the degree of autonomy and self-determination among individual people and in communities in order to enable them to represent their interests in a responsible and self-determined way, acting on their own authority, as detailed earlier [16]. It is the process of becoming stronger and more confident, especially in controlling one's own life and claiming one's own rights. Empowerment as action refers both to the process of self-empowerment and to professional support of people, which enables them to overcome their sense of powerlessness and lack of influence, and to recognise and use their resources. So empowerment implies a transfer of power. If power is the ability to do something or act in a particular way, then transferring power implies transferring the ability to do something. In the context of our individual relationship with the welfare sector, this transfer of power or empowerment means accepting that each individual is given responsibility to take control of their own life – their health and welfare. This means giving and accepting greater personal responsibility and the maturity involved. This empowerment is never going to be a black or white choice; some individuals will be able to cope with much more responsibility for their own decisions and future, while others will continue to need ongoing support.

CONCLUSION

This chapter has described a primary care sector including both health and broader welfare services that operates as a learning system and which all of us as citizens are involved with as service users, customers and patients. The elements defining our relationship with the sector – from our own personal mastery, the team working and relationships involved between care providers and the discussions and dialogue involved in their work through to the extent to which we accept personal responsibility for our own health, and the place of personal autonomy, advocacy and empowerment. Essentially we have described a sector which seeks to support learning as a learning system and not restrict the learning to saying what it is about or for or with or by, but rather it is learning to enable, to support and to provide, a system which is able to adapt to change and to transform, to be fit for the future.

Of course this learning system cannot be self-supporting. It has to evolve and thrive within a sector which is designed to be fit for purpose and commissioned to meet its responsibilities. This has to mean reconsideration of the organisational formats and business models in the sector and the way the sector is contracted or commissioned to perform. Until now, the professional partnership model has been the predominant model in the sector, but the self-employed, independent contractor model is no longer fit for purpose. Many are choosing salaried status as employees, and perhaps we need to enfranchise this choice to make it a legitimate career choice for clinicians of all disciplines. In addition we will need to look again at commissioning arrangements in the sector. National contacts for services such as the general medical services (GMS) and personal medical services (PMS) contracts for general medical practice lack the flexibility to respond to local circumstance and, as the CQC program has found, to nurture a culture of quality improvement or ensure safe care. At the same time, the alternative of shorter-term alternative provider medical services (APMS) contracting arrangements has not been shown to be an effective mechanism to drive quality improvement. The lack of any national or local body or system with responsibility for quality improvement in the sector is a concern, as is the lack of any option for local development planning to drive services towards local needs. Perhaps development plans derived from CQC reports could support locality commissioning and transformation towards the *practice at scale* being trialled though the *Five Year Forward View* Vanguard projects [14].

REFERENCES

1. Starey N, Bosanquet N and Griffiths J. 1993. General practitioners in partnership with management: An organisational model for debate. *BMJ* 306:308–10.
2. Senge PM. 1990. *The Fifth Discipline.* Currency/Doubleday, New York.
3. 16 Personality Types. 2019. www.personalityperfect.com/16 personality-types.
4. Fisher SG, Hunter TA and Macrosson WDK. 1998. The structure of Belbin's team roles. *J Occup Organ Psychol* 71:283–8.
5. The Victoria Climbie inquiry: Report of an inquiry by Lord Laming. 2003. TSO, London.
6. West MA. 2003. *Effective Teamwork: Practical Lessons from Organizational Research. Illusions of Teamworking in Healthcare 2013 and Why Teamwork Matters 2013.* BPS Blackwell, Malden, MA.
7. Royal College of General Practitioners (RCPG). RCGP toolkit for substance misuse 2004. https://www.rcgp.org.uk/learning/substance-misuse-and-associated-health-landing-page.aspx.
8. Bohm dialogue. 2019. http://www.david-bohm.net/dialogue/.
9. Schon D. 1983. *The Reflective Practitioner: How Professionals Think in Action.* Basic Books, New York.
10. Starey N. 2003. *The Challenge for Primary Care.* Radcliffe Press, Oxford, pp. 117–37.
11. Cream J, Maguire G and Robertson R. 2018. How have public attitudes to the NHS changed over the past three decades? https://www.kingsfund. org.uk/publications/how-have-public-attitudes-to-nhs-changed.
12. House of Commons Health Committee. 2016. Primary care: Fourth report of session 2015–16. HC 408. www.parliament.uk/healthcare.

13. Mele AR. 1995. *Autonomous Agents: From Self-Control to Autonomy.* Oxford University Press, Oxford.
14. NHS. New care models. https://www.england.nhs.uk/new-care-models/2015 accessed 2015.
15. Ham SC et al. 2018. https://www.kingsfund.org.uk/publications/shared-responsibility-health.
16. O'connor 2018. What does it mean to be an empowered patient. https://www.powerfulpatients.org.

7

Systems thinking in primary care "system archetypes"

INTRODUCTION

While the previous chapter explored the elements which together can promote a *culture* of learning, development and effective team working in the primary care sector, this chapter looks at *systems thinking* [4] as applied to the sector and explores some of the design features which affect the sector's ability to learn, develop and deliver better care.

Systems thinking (ST) is an approach to focussing on the whole process rather than individual bits or constituents – looking at films rather than still photos and plays rather than individual scenes. This is illustrated in Figure 7.1. The whole diagram represents the primary care system and it contains several areas or subdivisions.

This chapter and the next requires us to consider behaviour within the primary care sector and between it and other sectors in patterns, system archetypes, and also some designs or paradigms. Systems thinking requires us to put together all the elements making up the system so as to understand how they relate to each other and to appreciate the principles underpinning the systems performance.

To help us explore systems thinking in the National Health Service (NHS) primary care system we will use two analytical tools:

- Recognising archetypes
- The evolution of paradigms

But first we need to understand the difference between primary care as a sector and primary care as a system.

The primary care *sector* is that part of the British healthcare sector to which all UK citizens have direct access. It is our first point of contact and is characterised by, as we have discussed earlier (see Chapter 1),

- *Universal coverage*: The whole population from cradle to grave.
- *Generalist approach*: All health problems dealt with as opposed to segmented by emphasis on specialist care.

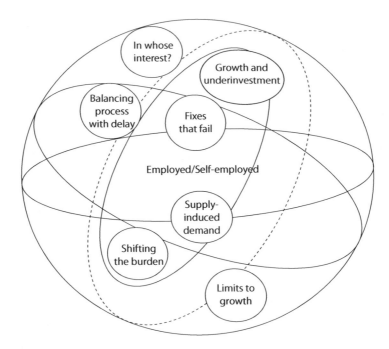

Figure 7.1 Primary care paradigms and archetypes.

- *Biographical care*: Registration and a lifelong medical record containing our health biography, informing our relationship with the sector.
- *Free to use at the point of need*: Not dependent on the user's ability to pay or insurance status.

If these characteristics are the sector's heritage, then adapting to the new digital future of the primary care sector is now essential if the sector is to remain relevant and retain is independence. We need to understand the pros and cons of the transformation that is entailed. The chair of NHS England, Prof Sir Malcolm Grant, has predicted the demise of the traditional GP model [1], but the report of a review into the model [2] presents a much more positive picture. The truth is that, if it is to survive, professional partnership as a business model will need to adapt to the realities of modern life. The digital world offers rapid access and convenience to the population with the internet enfranchising all those with access to it to all the products of the *information revolution*. But access to the data and information is not the same as knowing everything or being empowered to use the information, yet alone using it wisely. There is still a place for expertise in helping the population interpret information, individualising it and helping people interpret the information in the context of their life and supporting them in making decisions that are right for them. In inspecting digital providers [3] the Care Quality Commission (CQC) has found much to commend but also raised concerns about some aspects of safety such as ensuring each individual's identity, aspects of medicines management such as ensuring safe care of patients on high-risk medicines or accessing controlled drugs, and ensuring liaison with other services involved with providing care in line with guidance from other regulators and in ways that ensure the digital services can enhance patient care rather than confuse it.

These features make the NHS primary care sector unusual in the modern world and are the features which have underpinned the reputation of the whole NHS around the world. For instance, see the US Commonwealth Fund [4] comparison of international health system performance, which rates these key features highly. The sector is therefore the anatomy of primary care describing what the sector consists of while the primary care system refers to the design of the sector as its physiology, how and why it works efficiently, its cultures and its relationships:

- How it is put together
- How it works
- How it delivers care
- How it is managed
- How its internal and external relationships are organised
- How it learns and develops over time

This means looking at the context within which individuals and teams working in the sector operate and work together. It means looking at the attitudes, values and beliefs held within the primary care sector, and also at some of the forces which shape practitioners and other stakeholders as individuals and teams and how they are responding to the pressures they have to cope with.

To help us understand the sector and the system we will use examples of paradigms and archetypes. First, we need to define what we mean by them – and both of them are going to be needed to answer the what, the how and the why questions – involved in understanding the system.

- *Paradigms* are key features that characterise the sector. They are patterns or models which describe how the system is put together – the patterns which distinguish and characterise the sector and influence its performance. We shall look further at paradigms and their impact in the next chapter.
- *Archetypes* are recurring themes that we can learn to recognise and that underpin how all systems work, including the primary care system. These archetypes and examples of how they work in the primary care sector form most of the rest of this chapter.
  - They describe and determine how the system will respond to circumstances as they change, so we will consider how the system is responding to current circumstances.
  - They require us stop thinking in purely structural terms – the anatomy of the sector and the system – and start thinking dynamically, both in terms of time and in terms of relationships and interactions, physiology rather than anatomy.
  - They help us to understand and interpret why the system works the way it does. Why cherry-picking by digital providers is a current battleground is an example.

* Fundamentally, they help us to appreciate that systems work the way they do *because that is how they are designed to work*. If form is to follow function, then when functions need to change to meet a changing world or circumstance, then form has to respond if the system is to continue to work. So, as the functions of organisations and teams in the primary care sector evolve and change as care is provided at home rather than in hospital, so the team and organisational form needs to evolve and change to meet the new circumstances they face.
* An analogy from the education sector can help us by illustrating the use of the terms *system*, *sector*, *paradigm* and *archetype* as well as the importance of attitudes, values and beliefs in determining performance.

Helen was starting at secondary school. She felt well prepared, was happy and content, had done well at her primary school, and was going with many of her friends, and had a glowing report from her primary school headmistress. Helen knew the way to school, had visited it for a "transition" day, read about the school on its website and was keen to grab the opportunities which she knew were ahead.

What she did not realise was the extent to which the institution and culture of a large secondary school was going to affect her learning. The way in which disruptive children and overburdened teachers would make it difficult for her to learn, and the isolation and feeling of floundering that she was going to feel in a school that was some ten times larger than her primary school. She did not realise how pressurised her time was going to be, how much she was going to have to fit into and mould herself around the routine of school and homework, and the extent to which her success would be down to that spark of motivation and enthusiasm that she might or might not find.

In this analogy from the education sector, the comprehensive paradigm is the predominant form of provision in the secondary education sector. The archetypes Helen will experience, and which will hopefully enhance her learning, include the following:

* *Shifting the burden to the intervener*: The task of the school is seen as supporting Helen's learning rather than taking a "chalk and talk" approach to teaching her, or "ramming down her throat" what she needs to know. This is a shift to supporting student-centred learning, a shift in the locus of power from the provider (the teachers and school) to the recipient or student.
* *Escalation*: In the classroom context this so often leads to conflict and detention, as small disagreements or issues rapidly spiral out of control. It can also lead to sporting excellence, scholarship and leadership – one thing leads to another in either a vicious or virtuous cycle. In a school which has always excelled in science, for example, there is an inbuilt or cultural expectation that this will continue.
* *Eroding goals*: This is concentration on the short term and letting the long-term goals slip. It is so easy to concentrate on the exam or national curriculum, on mastering the techniques involved in science or mathematics at the expense of

mastering the principles and developing an understanding among the students of the reasons why it is important to study the issues at hand and read around the subject so as to provide a broader approach.

My maths master Mr T was a soldier in World War I who had been gassed and suffered from shell shock, which we would now recognise as post-traumatic shock disorder. He helped me scrape through O-level elementary maths by force-feeding me formulae and equations in a way that ensured I never understood the subject, how it had evolved, its links to other subjects and the contribution it makes to all aspects of life. On the other hand, Mr Tree, an early environmental activist who had a car with a "town gas bag" as a power source on its roof, helped me to an *A* grade in A-level biology by sparking my interest in genetics "alternation of generations" and the beauty of nature, membership of the British Society for Social Responsibility in Science, and an early appreciation of the causes and consequences of global warming. That spark is really important, but too often the goal is eroded and the spark dulled by the short-term focus on exams.

- *Success to the successful*: The teacher focusses on the top students in the class giving them extra time and encouragement, while the slower learners are left to struggle and flounder. Inevitably, as in all walks of life, this can be a recipe for fragmentation; disharmony; the rise of negativism; and the fertile soil in which radical ideas such as fascism, populism and religious fanaticism can germinate and flourish. On the other hand, it is also the archetype which promotes excellence – scholarship, gold medals and elitism.
- *Fixes that fail*: Too much focus on short term or quick fixes at the expense of their long-term consequences. It is sometimes easier to rigidly enforce a uniform rule about social media or IT use rather than evolving a framework to encourage a mature and balanced approach to personal appearance and behaviour in a community with a wide range of values and norms. This promotion of maturity is tricky. Young people in the secondary school will mature physically, mentally and emotionally at different rates and times, so boundaries and goals will need to be agreed and set. But promoting personal responsibility and a sense of being valued as a person are really important. It is a fundamental theme of this book that such maturity is required and needs promoting if the goal of *promoting the welfare of the population* is to be realised.

Each of these, and others which Helen will come across, will not be explicitly described and manipulated during her time at the school, but they are underlying descriptors of the "way the system works" which will affect her life at school.

If we return to consider how the system works in the primary care sector of the NHS, then we can better appreciate the key common design features between the education and health systems.

- *Shifting the burden to the intervener archetype*: A key feature of the work of Illich's writing [5,6] is the damaging effect that *professional capture* has on the product that is a key feature, so that teachers may inhibit learning and doctors may be bad for health. If shifting the burden in the education world means supporting learning, then in the primary healthcare system it means empowering patients, or the users of the system, to improve their own health by taking personal responsibility for it. In the first seventy years of the NHS the "burden" has been borne by healthcare professionals, that is, doctors, nurses, and so on, who have the power (basically the ability and knowledge to do something, make it happen) to make decisions about or on behalf of any individual in their care and about aspects of their healthcare. Shifting the burden or responsibility to the intervener means freeing patients from their position of being the recipient of healthcare towards being partners in the search for solutions to the health issues they face, be it the genes they carry, the infection they have caught or the long-term condition they develop (diabetes, asthma or hypertension for example). An example of this archetype in action is the approach to smoking cessation where individuals have been supported to stop smoking with a range of interventions – from economic to pharmaceutical – but it is the individual who has to struggle with the withdrawal from nicotine dependence involved and reap the rewards in terms of health benefit is theirs. It has been one of the great public health successes of the last twenty years that the rate of smoking in England has halved – to between sixteen percent and seventeen percent – and it has happened by a strategic approach that has included taxation, legislation, culture and persuasion. But it would not have worked if this archetype had been ignored. Such an approach to patient empowerment, "shifting the burden" has not been a prominent feature of the findings of the CQC from its inspection programme in the sector [7], but one example would be [8] where for the last twenty years the drive has been to shift the burden in this way. The resulting savings – reduced resource utilisation year-on-year – are in stark contrast to the rest of the sector's experience of rising demand and falling profitability. So, one of the key planks of the transformation programme this book recommends is adoption, systematically, of this archetype in the primary care sector: to empower individual citizens to take on responsibility for their own health. To adopt policies and approaches which learn from our experience of adopting seat belts in our cars, moving away from addiction to nicotine, and towards active citizenship [7,9], which has largely been discussed in terms of the education sector but deserves wider attention in health. The new opportunities provided by universal access to the internet and all the information is offers enables not only convenience and expertise to be available at the click of a mouse but also offers the opportunity to liberate the population from the repressive yoke of *professional capture*.

Moving beyond the individual citizen, communitarianism has been a feature of some CQC inspections of "outstanding" general practices in England where the strong links between the organisation and the community – be it local authority, employers or third-sector organisations – have been features which have empowered citizens to enrich their lives and move beyond being passive recipients of healthcare.

- *Escalation*: In the consulting room, the differing perspectives and attitudes of the people involved can trap them into behaviour which, in the end, can cause problems for each. This example involves both escalation and elements of *eroding goals and shifting the burden* archetypes but is really important as it shows what a terrible position people, both providers of care and those seeking care, can end up in.

A specialist private clinic in Sheffield helps people with long-term addiction problems by inserting naltrexone implants to reduce cravings for both opiate- and alcohol-dependent situations. The doctor is a long-retired GP with experience in the field, but he is isolated from peer support and is providing an unsafe service using an unlicensed product. Pressure from users of his service is the main reason why the service has continued, and this pressure has increased or escalated as other treatment options have reduced as providers have withdrawn from treatment provision, to the extent that he cannot even pick his raspberries in peace in his garden without interruption from desperate individuals pleading for help. We have to reflect that opiate and alcohol addiction is a major factor behind acquisitive crime, is a major problem for the prison service, destroys the lives of individual and their families, and is associated with long-term health problems and a cycle of deprivation, abuse and violence. At the same time, sufferers feel victimised and feel that they are out of control and unable to take any responsibility for their situation. Rather they escalate the issue by blaming everyone else for their situation, antagonising those trying to help them. In addition the *escalation* spiral is tightened by development of complex co-morbidities – both mental and physical – leading to a greatly reduced life expectancy; complex psychopathology; a range of safeguarding problems affecting them, their children and their families; and a drift into criminal behaviour and marginalisation from membership in society.

Until we see this issue as an example of systemic failure and develop a holistic, strategic response as a community and society, this problem of addiction will grow; destroy lives, families and communities and consume more and more resources. It is in nobody's interest that this continues, but we are all "blind" – *there is none so blind as those who will not see* [10].

- *Supply-induced demand*: This is one of a small number of recurring patterns of structure, or system archetypes, which between them form the key to understanding and interpreting any system. Between them, these archetypes suggest that management problems are never unique – something experienced managers know intuitively. If homeostasis, servomechanisms and leverage are the basic tools of systems thinking, then system archetypes are analogous to the stories that get told over and over again. The same archetypes occur in a variety of different sectors – economics, politics, science, business and healthcare. It is understanding and using them which makes systems thinking such a powerful tool. Because archetypes are subtle, we may not recognise them when we first see them. Sometimes they produce a sense of déjà vu, but often it can be sometime later and following a period of reflection that we realise what we are dealing with.

In the supermarket world, increasing the demand for a product can be stimulated by increasing its availability – piling high and selling cheap, sells everything from soap powder to breakfast cereals in the short term. But just as Senge [4] describes *growth and underinvestment*, this archetype only works in the longer term if capacity enhancement is tackled by investment, training, education and relationship management. So in healthcare, setting targets is almost bound to fail because it simply stimulates demand without addressing the systems capacity. In primary care, fuelling demand for additional access to GP or dental appointments leads to inefficient use of scarce professional resources. Stimulating demand without increasing supply does not work and leads to poor quality of care. The CQC inspection programme in English general practice found too many examples of practices where access to appointments was problematic. This fuelled poor performance and poor quality of care. Detailed in the *National GP Patient Survey* and poor feedback on *NHS Choices* [11], these practices and their commissioners had failed to understand the system archetype, that is, supply-induced demand or growth and underinvestment produces poor performance and system "stress" often leading to system failure, an "inadequate" CQC rating and provider failure. The solution needs to be a more systematic approach to understanding the drivers of the demand/supply mismatch and addressing them through investment, training, education and effective commissioning, and in particular by paying attention to empowering people to have more control over their own lives and the service they are trying to access. Individual citizens need the opportunity to learn how to use the service in mature ways, to take responsibility for their own health and to make adult choices about their healthcare needs or their welfare. The current approach to dealing with provider failure, by relying on short-term alternative provider medical services (APMS) contracting arrangements through a range of private sector providers, seems to be a recipe for continued provider failure, burnout of provider clinicians and poor care for local people. This is an example – alongside other archetypes like *fixes that fail*, *tragedy of the commons* and *success to the successful* – where two-dimensional thinking or simply dealing with the presenting symptoms is not enough. Rather a more holistic approach, or an approach that considers the cause of the symptoms, is required. This approach asks why is the system behaving the way it is and uses this analysis to design solutions. Until the primary care sector adopts this approach, designed and commissioned in a way which draws on such an analysis of the symptoms and problems it is facing, it seems it is likely to continue to struggle. General medical services (GMS), personal medical services (PMS) and APMS contracts for GP services alongside the national dental, pharmaceutical and optical contracts have remained the cornerstone of the relationship between independent contractors and the NHS throughout the last seventy years, but are no longer sufficiently flexible to adapt to the varying circumstances local providers are experiencing.

My clinical work in recent years has mostly been in the urgent care sector as a doctor for the out-of-hours service. It has become apparent that this "supply-induced demand" archetype is thriving in this sector because of the isolation of the subunits in the primary care sector. The subunits I am referring to include local general medical practices; other urgent care sector providers such as walk-in centres, the ambulance service and hospital accident and emergency (A&E) departments; social care providers such as nursing and care homes; local dental providers; local pharmacies; and mental health teams. The police and fire services also get caught up in the archetype occasionally. It all goes wrong when subunits are either not effectively communicating with each other or are shifting the burden of responsibility around the sector without realising the consequences. Over a recent Christmas period, the GP out-of-hours service was as busy as it had planned to be, based on previous years experience. But recent pressure on local general practices [12] seems to have affected the behaviour of local people. Whereas in previous years the phone system was requiring doctors to call people back about health problems and would have over a hundred calls logged at any one time, recently the numbers have been consistently over 200. Talking to colleagues about their experience and the reasons for it clarified that people were calling the out-of-hours service because of difficulty getting appointments at their usual GP surgery during working hours. Colleagues felt that lack of coordination was leading to people using the service differently and in a way that the service was struggling to cope with. At present the urgent care sector struggles to be an effective partner in the local health economy because links with NHS 111 and other urgent care providers are weak. Even the nurses working in our local minor injury unit tell me that they lack any sense of belonging to a coordinated and coherent service; there is a lack of a common health record so that people using the service often have to repeat their story several times; transfer arrangement when people's needs require it are inefficient and often time-consuming; and links with other sectors, like social services, hospitals and mental health teams, are too reliant on personal relationships rather than effective systems with fallback safety nets. The result is disjointed service provision despite the best of intentions.

- *Tragedy of the commons*: First identified by ecologists, it describes what happens when what is right for each local part of the system is wrong for the whole. The archetype is useful for dealing directly with problems where apparently logical decision making can become completely illogical for the larger system.

For example, the Sahel region in sub-Saharan Africa was once a fertile pastureland. In the middle of the twentieth century it supported over a hundred thousand herdsmen and over half a million head of grazing cattle (the zebu). Today, it is a barren desert, yielding a small fraction of the vegetation it produced before. The people left there scratch out a meagre existence under the continual threat of drought and starvation.

The tragedy was rooted in the steady growth of population and herd sizes from the 1920s to the 1970s. Aid and unusually heavy rains incentivised the expansion of the herds due to each herdsman deciding to keep more zebu for economic gain and social status. In the early 1960s, overgrazing began to occur and vegetation became sparser leading to overgrazing and eventually desertification. This became a vicious spiral of decline until a series of droughts in the 1960s and 1970s. By the early 1970s, fifty to eighty percent of the livestock was dead and much of the population was destitute. The same story has been repeated all over the world in farmlands and rain forests where the logic of local decision making leads inexorably to the "common" resource depletion and to overexploitation and ends in tragedy. In the primary care sector, each individual practice, pharmacy shop and family makes decisions about what is right for them. But each decision has resource implications for the rest of the sector and the community, and in the end can lead to tragedy because they focus on what is right for them, not on the needs of the whole.

In the primary care sector, this archetype shows itself in the issue of antibiotic resistance and the rise of associated health problems. Over the first seventy years of the NHS a whole range of effective antibiotics have been developed and as a result, alongside other developments such as immunisation and education, the *five giants* (see Chapter 3) have been in retreat. However, local decision making, by every prescriber and every patient requesting antibiotics, risks the *common good*. Who manages the commons is as much an issue in the NHS as it is in sub-Saharan Africa. The tragedy of desertification and population destitution could be repeated unless we learn to manage the commons – multiresistant TB, the rise of *Clostridium difficile* and of methicillin-resistant *Staphylococcus aureus* can only reinforce the need for effective control.

The issue of localness and its management alongside the management of the commons is also important in the primary care sector. An issue that has arisen several times during the recent CQC inspection programme in general practice [7] has been the difficulty that distant, national provider organisations have experienced when dealing with and supporting small local practices. The local practice will frequently have long experience of autonomy – making its own decisions without considering the effect on the wider community. Now, as part of a larger corporate community of primary care units (often including walk-in centres, and new APMS practices for special populations such as students, the homeless or refugees) they find that the corporate provider does not give them the support and attention that they feel they need to meet their needs. In this situation the "commons" is the interest of the whole community served by the larger, corporate provider, and the tragedy is that the provider often struggles to meet both the local interests and those of the wider community. All for one and one for all can be difficult to hold together and CQC has certainly found examples of the tensions involved. In looking at this archetype it is all too easy to sympathise with the herdsman/local provider/antibiotic seeker, but one of the founding distinguishing features of the NHS is its universality – one for all and all for one. Perhaps bridging the gap between local decision making and the broader community interest requires consideration of the paradigms involved.

PARADIGMS

This brings us to consider the place and evolution of paradigms within the primary care sector. While the predominant paradigm over the last seventy years has been the *medical model*, there is a strong argument for it to adapt to change by morphing a *reductionist* approach into a more *holistic biopsychosocial* model [13].

However, there is a need for a reconsideration, not just of the way we classify and treat illness but also of the way we organise the provision of care to take account of the new realities and possibilities opened up by the digital age and the more mature relationships between care providers and care receivers that we have been considering.

Features of the medical model in the NHS during the last seventy years

- An anatomical approach to managing care – making a diagnosis by taking the patient's history, a physical examination of the patient, and considering the results of tests and arranging interventions or treatments. Along with a scientific element to ensure learning from success and a refining treatment as appropriate.
- Doctor knows best – with supplicant patients waiting for care, and powerful professionals determining provision.
- Specialist care in hospitals – either as inpatients in beds or through day care or outpatient clinics. Attempts to move specialist care into the community have mostly been limited to specialities treating people in their own home, for example dermatology, elderly care and mental health. Hospitals mainly provide treatment for an episode of care, not usually having continuing responsibility for the care of the patient beyond that "episode". Continuing attendance at outpatients following an inpatient episode of care is a particular feature of the NHS. Much more specialist follow-up occurs than in other healthcare systems, but the degree does vary from area to area and between specialities. Canada cares for widely scattered populations, so its adoption of digital follow-up is perhaps unsurprising but something we could learn from.
- Expert generalist care outside hospital – provided by general practitioners and their employed teams alongside community staff such as district nurses. Characteristics of this home-based, expert generalist care include *registration* (everybody registering for care with a GP surgery), *universal coverage of the whole population*, and *continuing responsibility for care* (while both healthy and when sick, so-called *biographical care*).
- Transfer between generalist and specialist care by a system of referral – traditionally between GP and consultant with letters copied to patients. This gatekeeping with the GP and consultant regulating access to care now seems outdated. It does little to promote shifting the burden to the intervenor and promotes the culture of medical model control and restricts the power of other professionals to access and discharge patients efficiently.
- Nursing and other professions allied to medicine are supportive of this medical model and are not offering an alternative paradigm.

However, the medical model, as a paradigm, cannot be considered in isolation from other paradigms that are features of current life in the UK. We live in a welfare state where benefits such as primary and secondary education, unemployment pay, social security sickness pay and pensions are universal. Each of these paradigms has evolved since the introduction of the welfare state in the middle of the last century. There are many attractive features of life in the welfare state:

- Lifelong support for all citizens. No matter what life might throw at us, we can always rely on the welfare state.
- No need to look to our savings to pay for our children's education or to fund health bills or periods of unemployment.
- Security in old age with an old age pension.

There are also significant disadvantages:

- A culture of dependency rather than self-reliance. If we can rely on the state, perhaps we don't need to protect ourselves or invest in our own future development or make provision for our own family's welfare.
- While healthcare is provided, free at the point of need, social care is not. People needing social care, for example in old age, have to pay for it. This has been an increasing burden for many in recent years and has led to many family homes being sold to fund social care. A government green paper is awaited to describe options for the future, but if any resolution was easy or simple we would have found it years ago [14].
- In our modern materialistic society we may not truly value the cheap product, and when healthcare is free at the point of use, perhaps the value of it is underappreciated. As the cost of the NHS grows at an inexorably faster rate than inflation, it is easy to feel that individual citizens are entitled to everything it can provide, rather than only look to it for vital necessities. Cosmetic products, dietary supplements and baby milks are examples where the culture of entitlement has been questioned at times. Little attention has been given to informing people using NHS services of the cost of the service or helping them understand the cost effectiveness of the proposed intervention or of the choices open to them.

Perhaps the medical model Mk 2 or any new paradigm underpinning the design of the primary care sector has to move the culture of "medical" towards "welfare", recognising that the paradigm cannot be narrowly restricted and perhaps it also needs to bring community, financial, employment and education within a "big tent" paradigm. It is also increasingly apparent that current paradigms ignore issues of mature behaviour at their peril. Just as in the education example, pupil uniform and behaviour rules might benefit from an understanding of what drives mature and immature behaviour, so in the move from a medical paradigm to a welfare paradigm we will need to ensure that incentives for more mature behaviour are designed in. In the next chapter, we will consider paradigms further as we move towards the final section of this book, and the elements required to redesign the primary care sector to make it fit for purpose in the modern, digital world.

REFERENCES

1. Bower E. 2018. Traditional GP model will be swept aside by tech revolution, NHS England chair predicts. *GP Online*, June 28. https://www.gponline.com/traditional-gp-model-will-swept-aside-tech-revolution-nhs-england-chair-predicts/article/1486311.
2. Watson N. 2018. *GP Partnership Review: Interim Report*. NHSE, London.
3. Care Quality Commission. 2018. The state of care in independent online primary health services. https://www.cqc.org.uk/sites/default/files/20180322_state-of-care-independent-online-primary-health-services.pdf.
4. Senge PM. 1990. *The Fifth Discipline*. Currency/Doubleday, New York.
5. Illich I. 1975. *Limits to Medicine: Medical Nemesis; The Expropriation of Health*. Penguin, London.
6. Illich I. 1971. *Deschooling Society*. Harper & Row, New York.
7. Care Quality Commission. 2017. *The State of Care in General Practice 2014–2017*. CQC, London.
8. The Old Dispensary Medical Practice. 2016. www.theolddispensary.co.uk.
9. British Council. 2009. Active Citizens. https://www.britishcouncil.org/active-citizens.
10. Chalkley T. 2009. A collection of the works of Thomas Chalkley: In two parts. Text Creation Partnership and University of Oxford. http://tei.it.ox.ac.uk/tcp/Texts-HTML/free/N05/N05022.html.
11. www.gov.uk/NHS choices framework. January 2020.
12. Fletcher E, Abel GA, Anderson R et al. 2017. Quitting patient care and career break intentions among general practitioners in South West England: Findings of a census survey of general practitioners. *BMJ Open* 7:015853.
13. Introduction to health psychology. Lumen Boundless Psychology. https://courses.lumenlearning.com/boundless-psychology/chapter/introduction-to-health-psychology accessed on 31 January 2020.
14. Commission on the Future of Health and Social Care in England. 2014. A new settlement for health and social care: Final report [Barker Report]. The King's Fund, London. https://www.kingsfund.org.uk/sites/default/files/field/field_publication_file/Commission%20Final%20%20interactive.pdf.

8

Mutuality

INTRODUCTION

In bringing this part of the book concerning *analysis and interpretation* to an end, we need to bring several themes discussed earlier together, so that they can form parts of a coherent vision for the future of the primary care sector which is outlined in the final section in Chapters 9 and 10. These themes encompass the evolution of current *paradigms* to ensure they remain in line within the needs and views of the population in the modern world. It will become apparent that *system archetypes* as well as *paradigms* have to be considered. In using the tools of *systems thinking* they are equally important. The issue of mutual dependency or *mutuality* as it relates to the relationships between individuals and stakeholders within in the sector and beyond needs outlining as do some aspects of the *governance* of the sector to ensure that public confidence in the sector and its trustworthiness is assured, including aspects of the sectors provision which are funded from general taxation and those privately funded.

The end of the previous chapter outlined features that have made the "medical model" the predominant paradigm of the primary care sector during the last seventy years. In reality this paradigm is really a *professional rather than simply a medical model*. The whole physiology of the sector is based on the relationship between professionals and citizens, and driven by a culture and set of values which describe a view of professionalism. All the clinical professions involved in providing care in the sector have been part of this medical model or "professional paradigm". The roots of this model of "professionalism" stretch back into history (see Chapter 3) but need to be refreshed in this digital world of universal access to data and information; the more mature, educated and empowered citizen; and the requirement on all professionals (from clergy to solicitors, teachers and bankers) to be more open and transparent about their performance and more accountable to the people they serve and to the general public.

Vignette 1

I interviewed Molly a year or so ago, after hearing about her from her daughter, who had discussed this book project with her mother and knew Molly wanted to talk to me. Molly was in her eighties and had been receiving treatment for advanced cancer, but that had now finished. She was full of praise for the National Health Service (NHS) care she had received from her GP and his team who had looked after her for over thirty years, been there whenever she needed them, diagnosed her cancer and referred her for specialist treatment. However, she told me that they had never consulted her about her views of what aspects of their service could be improved about what could be done to actively involve her when planning her care. She was also indebted to the specialist team at the local hospital and to the hospice that had planned her care over recent weeks.

Molly had read about Dame Tessa Jowell's recent brain cancer treatment and her speech to the House of Lords [1] and read an essay by Tessa Richards in the *BMJ* [2]. Molly felt grateful to them for helping her understand that she needed to take a more active part in her cancer journey. Being the passive recipient of care had been OK all her life, and when she knew and trusted her professional team of advisers she felt confident enough to accept their plans – but this was no longer enough. She now felt that she deserved to have a voice and it needed to be heard. She wanted to share control over her life and did not want any further active treatment for her cancer. She wanted to be cared for at home in a way which respected her life's experience, her career as an academic leader in a world-class university, and as a mother, grandmother and great grandmother. She wanted her doctor (GP) to be her clinical representative and to take her views to the local multidisciplinary team meeting at the hospital and the palliative care meeting at the practice, and to link through her daughter, who held her lasting power of attorney, to the rest of the family. Molly told me that she now felt that there were aspects of "professionalism" that she had experienced that moved beyond benign "paternalism" towards "abusive, coercive control", and this worried her a great deal. "I think more vulnerable people would find some of the 'professional' behaviour and attitudes quite degrading, and I am ashamed that I did not challenge it".

Molly ended her interview by thanking me for taking the trouble to seek her out, listening to her and made me promise to publish this note of her views. Molly died in March 2018.

FROM THE PROFESSIONAL PARADIGM TO MUTUALITY

Common parlance speaks of paradigms shifting, a bit like tectonic plates moving at times leading to earthquakes. But the reality is that these changes are usually a bit more gradual – more evolution than revolution – and happen over time as a result of pressures on the current paradigm. The predominant professional paradigms in the NHS are being influenced by

- The enfranchisement of individual citizens – universal education meaning a more inquisitive population, access to information via the internet meaning a better informed population and increasing leisure and early retirement – so with more time to be involved with their own and their family's care.
- The decline in the role of "vocation" as a driver of professional life – those involved put more importance on a work–life balance than earlier generations did. The diversity and cultural mix in all the professions has meant that a much more diverse set of values is supporting professional practice. For my parents' generation, religious faith was a powerful foundation of vocation [3], but cultural diversity in the clinical professions has exposed the population to many different versions and degrees of vocation. I have met and worked closely with clinicians from India, Pakistan, Turkey, Poland, Ireland, Iraq and the USA, and interviewed an even greater range on Care Quality Commission (CQC) business. Across the range I have met hugely committed professionals, all working within the NHS for an ideal they share – universal healthcare, available to all, free at the point of need. They all share the desire for this to be available in the countries of their birth but have stayed working in the NHS – often for many years – to give them and their family a better life. However, there is no doubt in my mind and experience that their vocation has its roots in their own cultural background. For example, family input into care of the sick is much more a feature in India and Pakistan than in England, and our well-developed professional nursing system is in contrast to many other countries where the family provides all the personal care.
- The culture of deference, which lies behind Molly's acceptance of her role as a dependent patient, is no longer as dominant as it was in the early years of the NHS. Now we all complain at will – or give negative feedback on TripAdvisor – when we think we have been wronged. The compensation culture is rife and we will change our booking, our children's school, GP, bank or electricity provider much more easily than our parents would. Fear of "comeback" is still there but less dominant. We now consider it our right to have our own choice of service provider and to challenge their position whenever we want.

What seems to be emerging is a relationship between users of a service and providers based on a new balance of rights and responsibilities. There is an acceptance that "expertise" is useful as a guide to choice, but that ultimately it is the service user who is in control. "It's my money or my child or my holiday and I will decide what I am going to do". In the NHS this change in relationships needs acknowledging and is a pressure or influence on the professional paradigm. Some twenty years ago, while reflecting on the problem of delivering a transformation programme through a traditional GP partnership-run practice [4], I suggested a model for an organisation based on "mutuality". While the passage of time has made much of this thinking past its sell-by date, the underlying issue remains relevant: the current predominant organisational form in the primary healthcare sector, the GP partnership, and it needs to adapt and change if it is to remain fit for purpose. The modern world requires a rebalancing of stakeholder powers, a new relationship which reflects the enfranchisement of people registered with the practice, the expertise of clinicians providing advice and care within the organisation, and the interest of the broader community in establishing an organisation that can be trusted by all the stakeholders, be accountable for its performance and use of resources, and open to outside scrutiny. The organisation needs to be efficiently and sensitively led and managed in ways which respect and value staff and stakeholders alike. This kind of organisation is found in other sectors where it is seen that the mutual interest of all the parties involved is to support it. Perhaps the most obvious example is the traditional building society, where the savings of many individuals are used to provide loans (mortgages) for those buying property. The wages of staff and other costs of running the society are covered from the savings. In recent years, demutualisation or corporatisation of the mortgage supply business has meant payouts for investors, just as privatisation has done in other public service providers, but the cooperative movement, the strong third sector and the housing association movement remain as examples of community interest organisations which the primary care sector could and should and indeed has been looking to models for supporting this process of organisational evolution. This implies that the predominant paradigm is evolving towards a mutuality model. The CQC has inspected some excellent examples of this kind of organisation [5]; but they are unusual and exceptional examples that others might learn from.

In considering the emergence of this mutuality paradigm we also need to consider and include two other parts of the primary care sector which citizens use as *first point of contact* when they have healthcare needs:

1. *The urgent care sector*: Including walk-in centres, GP out-of-hours services and also perhaps NHS minor injury units. The complexity of the system through which citizens access and receive care in the "urgent care sector" and the consequent development of triage arrangements such as NHS 111 needs to be simplified and bought together as an integrated coherent system to become part of the mutuality paradigm.

Vignette 2

I saw Michael one night as the last patient on my list for the GP out-of-hours shift. He had metastatic cancer and needed help. Discharged from hospital in the last few days he is being looked after at home by his wife and family with input from community nurses, the local hospice team and his GP. Over the weekend he had become more frail, more breathless, found eating and drinking too exhausting, and had been struggling to stand and move to the bathroom. The GP out-of-hours service was very stretched. There were not enough doctors to man the home visiting service adequately and a constant backlog of over 100 calls waiting to be called back and triaged. I visited

Michael and arranged his admission for a further transfusion, but that is not the issue. We need an urgent care system which is fit for purpose "by design" – that can ensure that it is safe for Michael and his family, one they can trust, know that his care will not require me to intervene and "make decisions" – because the current system is failing. The GP out-of-hours system needs to "design in" the kind of capacity and escalation arrangements which help other emergency services to cope with fluctuating demand, the coastguard and lifeboats for example. The resilience of the urgent care sector requires layers of protection to protect the services from overload and failure. Additional triage and clinical capacity can be mobilised when required from trained clinicians working digitally from home and from the rest of the primary care sector to offer support as part of mutuality arrangements.

I supported a CQC inspection of a walk-in centre in Bracknell. This was provided by a distant national corporate provider as part of a government initiative to "support" struggling GP practices in the area and provide additional primary care capacity for people who found access to their GP was inadequate to meet their needs. The centre was not adequately staffed, the systems through which the centre and the care it provided were managed were dysfunctional, and the support from the corporate provider was unreliable. Just another example where a failure of mutuality was leading to people receiving poor care despite the best of intentions of all the stakeholders.

2. *Digital sector*: Including those providing support to the medicines supply arrangements – (community pharmacy and dispensing doctors) and those directly providing clinical services. Most of these providers are in the independent or private sector, and charge users a fee either for service or through subscription arrangements. In the main these services are provided for an episode of care rather than in support of any kind of biographical, ongoing, relationship between the service and its customer. The CQC's inspection programme has found providers to be offering, mainly, quick access to customers and heard good feedback from them about the quality of service they provide. But the CQC also uncovered some unsafe practices, such as weaknesses in confirming individual's identity or safeguarding arrangements for children and vulnerable adults, and poor arrangements for ensuring coordination of care between the NHS and themselves. While following GMC guidance [6] to only send details of the care provided to the NHS GP practice with patient-informed consent, this was only complied in a minority of cases. This discoordination in the provision of care to people seeking advice or treatment can be harmful – either to the individual receiving treatment or to their future ongoing care.

Vignette 3

I was told about Andy: Aged thirty-eight, he is an airline steward but had a bad back. He wanted some painkillers before he went on a long-haul trip. He got a private script for a codeine and paracetamol product, but his GP was not informed. This was unfortunate because his GP records showed that he had reacted badly to codeine-based products in the past when he had an operation for impacted wisdom teeth. Andy became ill during his trip and was admitted to hospital for treatment following a bad reaction to codeine. He was facing a bill for several thousand pounds for hospital treatment.

What would seem to be required is a move from the current professional paradigm to a mutuality one where NHS (Mk 2) offers digital, urgent care and existing primary care services through one NHS (Mk 2) organisation established as a mutual organisation for the benefit of the population. In the same way as I propose the digital and urgent care sector's incorporation into this model, so the issue of the social care sector needs inclusion. This does not mean that all residential and nursing homes need to be taken over and managed by NHS (Mk 2) or that local authority social service departments should become part of the national welfare service. But we do need to design our welfare system better, in a way that designs in quality of care when we are elderly, weak and vulnerable, and empowers people and their families rather than disempowers them.

I envisage a mutual benefit organisation emerging from the GP at scale arrangements announced in the 2019 GP contract. The primary care network should encompass urgent care and digital provision within the NHS and also have responsibility for commissioning social care provision.

THE PRIMARY HEALTHCARE TEAM: TEAM WORKING

The 1966 GP charter negotiated between the Labour government and the British Medical Association's General Medical Services Committee (GMSC) (see Chapter 3) sparked the expansion of general practice from single-handed medical practitioners working in isolation from their own homes into group practices with nursing and ancillary support. These groupings formed the foundations of primary healthcare teams and were often joined by other clinicians caring for the local population in their own homes, such as district nurses, health visitors and midwives.

Michael West [7] has led research into the effectiveness of *team working* and his message is compelling:

Team working is the next area I want to talk about as we begin to look at how we can integrate health and social care then we need to develop really effective ways of working in teams and we know that team work in general is really good in health care and in the NHS, in the staff survey, the data we have shown that 91 percent of staff say that they work in a team and that feels great cause for celebration and then we asked three groups, across organisational and sector boundaries, some less simple questions. "Does your team have clear objectives?" Because that is the best predictor of performance in teams we found in the NHS and outside the NHS as well. "Do you work closely together to achieve those objectives and work as a team?" and "Do you meet regularly to review your performance and how it can be improved?" And we think those are kind of core conditions for what teamwork is about so if you apply those core conditions there is only about 40 per cent or slightly more, maybe 41 per cent, of people in the NHS who work in what we would call a real team. So we have got about nine per cent of people who say they *don't work in a team, about 40 per cent of people who we think what we would call real teams and about 50 per cent who say they work in a team but we think there are in a pseudo team.*

This is some data from a primary care trust showing the relationship between real team working, pseudo team working and organisational health and safety, and what it shows is that the more people working in real teams the lower the levels of injuries to staff in the previous year, the lower the levels of potentially harmful errors that staff witness and the lower the levels of physical violence and bullying and harassment. The more people working in pseudo teams, the higher the levels of those things. The data suggests to us that real team working is associated with higher quality safer working and that pseudo team working in addition is associated with harm. You know the implications of this in terms of leadership are about we really need to make sure that when we talk about team working in the NHS that we are really clear about where is the team? Who is in it? What are the objectives of the team? And let's make sure we get these teams meeting together regularly. The data on mortality also indicate that the more people within the NHS working in real teams in primary care and the acute sector, the lower the levels of patient mortality and these figures here look pretty small, 5% more staff working in teams a 3% drop in mortality rate. That's 40 deaths per year in an acute hospital but if you multiply that 5% up to the 50% I'm saying working in pseudo teams then that figures goes up to 400 and if you multiply that by the number of acute trusts there are, let's say, 190 to 200, then these figures start to become pretty powerful in terms of the message that they send.

This is a little tricky to translate in the modern primary care sector of the NHS. Setting clear objectives and working closely together to achieve them is difficult when clinicians often prioritise principles of clinical autonomy and personal responsibility above those of team working and shared objectives. This is particularly an issue when "team members" are employed by different organisations that often have their own management pressures and different priorities. If the message in favour of teams is powerful and compelling, as opposed to pseudo-teams, then the lesson from the last fifty years in the sector is that

- Coordination of objectives.
- Working closely together.
- Using shared clinical records.
- Being managed in terms of clinical performance either within the team or by using external performance management tools, such as professional appraisal systems.
- Having an approach to individual annual performance review, which acknowledges and respects team membership as an important part of members work and values their contribution to the team as well as to their employing organisation.
- Moving beyond this to looking for teams to have a common employer/management framework is particularly important when dealing with issues such as care of the dying, newborns or when involvement with safeguarding issues is a key feature.
- During the recent CQC inspection programme in general practice [8], the weakness of team working in current practice was frequently described: practices that never saw their health visitor despite having children with safeguarding concerns on their books, not meeting regularly with their community and district nurses despite sharing their caseload of people with nursing needs at home, and too frequently general practitioners not meeting regularly with their employed staff and clinicians. Now that advertisements for general practitioners to work as salaried employees outnumber advertisements for GP partners (by about 4:1 when I last checked), the issue would seem to be becoming one of GP practice and team disintegration rather than integration.
- There are several other stakeholders who need to be considered as part of the evolving mutuality paradigm because their commonality of interest would benefit, and benefit from closer alliance, team working and integration with the sector. In addition, the system would work more efficiently and help to lower the boundaries to effective care currently emphasised by structural rigidities.
- Nursing and residential care homes, digital providers of primary care services and urgent care sector providers all share responsibility for the care of people who have hitherto been the responsibility of NHS primary care providers. Currently, there is no concept of commissioning services for a local population that takes into account their contribution, that looks to supporting training and recruitment, managing performance and developing joint care plans. There are many people who could benefit from a fresh look at some of these issues [9]. A shared record (with consent) seems a small step to take but is uncommon in the digital health sector and a less than predominant feature in nursing and care homes. Even sharing records between the GP practice and the GP out-of-hours provider has been far from straightforward until recently.

My father-in-law has been in a local care home for the last three years. When he went there he had had a series of falls – one where he broke his arm – and it had become apparent that he was not safe at home. He was known to have a heart valve problem and, as a result, was on medication to regulate his heart. Eventually, after 13 falls, the penny dropped and I managed to persuade the care home manager and the GP to refer him to the cardiologist at the local hospital. After several appointments and tests they finally agreed to fit him with a pacemaker – and he has had no more falls. This story does not seek to find any fault, but is included to highlight the importance of joint care planning, particularly for people are frail and vulnerable. This more joined-up approach is the key recommendation of the review of care for the frail elderly undertaken by the CQC in twenty local authority areas in the last year or so [9] and encompasses workforce planning, training, care standards, regulation and joint commissioning. There have been many reviews and reports about funding care for the frail elderly over the last forty years – for example the Barker Report [10] – and we are promised government proposals during 2020, but much could and should be done to meet the needs of this vulnerable group of people.

COMMISSIONING

1. If the paradigm evolution from professional to mutual is to receive any real impetus, it needs some traction from commissioning. For seventy years the primary care sector (Chapter 3) has been administered "at arm's length" and not really been considered as part of the centre of National Health Service. GPs are independent contractors, self-employed and contracted with the NHS to have responsibility for their registered list. This contract has been centrally negotiated between GP representatives and the NHS, but this has usually been a transactional process rather than a transformative one. It is still a Morris Minor with extras, not a Tesla. The paradigm evolution I envisage is therefore to promote an approach which refashions the relationship between the individual citizen and the health service in such a way as to ensure it is fit for the purpose of delivering their health needs.

2. With the majority of care being provided in the primary care sector (as we have often been told by the RCGP), then this should no longer be regarded as a marginal or peripheral venue to be consigned to a subservient position beside the preeminent position of the local acute hospital. What would seem to be required is a contracting or commissioning framework supporting the key changes in relationships we have been considering: *the empowered patient*; *the redefined professional*; *mutuality and organisational integration* (Chapters 1 and 10). To deliver this "Tesla" model will require some visionary leadership, which has been sadly lacking around the table in recent years. And perhaps there may be a need to delegate responsibility for delivering it externally. Certainly the framework will need to be sensitive to the varying health priorities of local people and therefore probably informed by local government's health and well-being arm; sensitive to the changing demography which the primary care sector is caring for and sensitive to the problems it has inherited, including recruitment and retention of clinicians, accessibility, marginalisation from "where the real work is done" – hospital. Rather care is provided in relative

isolation by small provider organisations which are now beginning to "work at scale" and to learn lessons from around the world [11]. The vicious cycle that the archetype "tragedy of the commons" represents (Chapter 7), with its analogy to desertification in sub-Saharan Africa, to antibiotic overuse and balancing the interests of localness within corporate organisations, does not need to be vicious. It could be transformed into a virtuous cycle through this process of redesign, transformation and commissioning.

3. Other sectors, including social services, hospital trusts and clinicians, voluntary sector organisations, local authorities and councils, and local employers. The primary care sector has important external partners and relationships which also need attention if the lessons from its heritage (see Chapter 3) are to be learned. In the past, people only ended up in hospital when they were referred by their GP. Now NHS 111 refers a third of its callers to accident and emergency (A&E), walk-in centres are often co-located with or close to A&E departments, and neither the consultant (in hospital) or the GP (at home) has overall responsibility for any patient's journey. Do we need a new host of "care coordinators" or a new approach to virtual team working using Skype? This is not the place to propose solutions, but simply to raise issues within a framework where solutions might be found.

Vignette 4

Four years ago my elderly aunt Fay, then 99 and now 103, fell at home and fractured her pelvis. I hold power of attorney for her, but was away and, against her wishes, she ended up in hospital. When I returned the consultant told me he could not discharge her. It was a team decision and the key player was the occupational therapist who needed to assess my aunt's ability to cope in her own home. My aunt took her own discharge against medical advice and has never been back. She remains on no regular medication and has a healthy disrespect for all doctors and nurses. She was a midwife and nurse for over fifty years and knows her own mind. The point is "responsibility" and power: We need to find a way to empower the individual citizen to take control, whenever possible, so that they don't become the victim of "institutional capture".

Another example kindly provided by a colleague:

I would like to share with you the experiences of my mother who was admitted to hospital on the 29th November 2018 and discharged on the 8th January 2019. I am her daughter and I have power of attorney.

My mother is 89, very frail with multiple co-morbidities and was living in her own home with a full care package. On the 29th November 2018 she was a bit wheezy when the carers went in to get her up. They called the GP but was told to ring 999. They contacted me and despite my best efforts and pleading I could not stop the GP and the paramedics deciding between them to admit her. She was admitted to the local acute hospital with a suspected chest infection. Within hours of her arrival she was assessed as medically fit and required only oral antibiotics for her suspected chest infection, but by that time she was caught up in the "system" which took over.

She spent the first 28 hours on a trolley, first in A&E and then in the MAU [medical assessment unit]. It was noisy and loud and lacked any semblance of comfort and dignity. My mother was tired, frightened and confused, and she was either on the trolley or placed in an unsuitable chair where she sat in considerable discomfort.

She then went to an acute medical ward where the staff set about treating anything 'medical' they could find. No one took a proper medical history, no one was interested in my mother's wishes, no one had any plans for enabling her to get back home and they lost her DNACPR [do not attempt CPR]. She was in hospital a total of 40 days.

At some point and without any consultation with the family, the SALT [speech and language therapy] team initiated pureed food because someone decided her swallowing wasn't 'right' – and in doing so they deprived her of the small pleasure of choosing something to eat. Communication with the ward was very difficult. We were often told to ring back later or the person we spoke to gave only vague information.

I was told that my mother needed an Integrated Care Assessment form to be completed so that she could be referred to the hospital's social services department and they would decide on a package of care. I signed my part of that form on Monday 3rd December, three days after her admission to the ward, and I was told that it would be sent to the social care team later that day. That didn't happen. The care agency and I then spent the next 30 days contacting the ward and the social care team daily to try and make progress. The care agency and I offered numerous dates for discharge none of which were possible because staff on the ward had failed to fill out the ICA form and send it to the right department. When challenged they blamed each other or gave us information that turned out not to be true.

On the 7th of January my mother was moved to a discharge ward as the nurse explained that there was pressure on the beds. The irony of this is that my mother could have been out of the hospital weeks before but for the sake of a single piece of paper.

At 7 pm on the 7th I was called by a nurse to discuss discharge. She wanted to know the code to the keypad at my mother's house. I was astonished. My mother is helpless and by this stage completely immobile. We had carefully synchronised her discharge for 12 noon on the 8th so that the carers, the manual handing assessor and I would be at the house to oversee her transfer. Despite repeated conversation with the ward, the nurse seemed unaware of the plan and was fully prepared to send my mother home in the morning to an empty house.

At 12:00 on the 8th I was at my mother's house along with the care team. At 12:45 I received a call from a nurse in the discharge lounge admitting they had forgotten to arrange transport and my mother was still in the hospital. By the time she arrived home the care team had gone.

When I unpacked her belongings, I discovered she had been sent home with someone else's clothes. She had a sealed medicines bag with her take-home medicine as expected. Next to that was a large bag of miscellaneous medicines, some in boxes, some just loose strips – none of which she was taking and some of which belonged to another patient. It looked as if someone had opened my mother's medicine locker and swept the contents into a bag and then put in a TTO bag belonging to another patient as well.

The day before my mother went into hospital last November she was able to walk from room to room using her frame, sit at her dining table and eat the meals she chose, play cards, have fish and chips if she wanted, walk to her sitting room and watch television, speak to her family on the phone every day, and enjoy having her hair done once a week. Yes, she was frail and getting weaker but we all worked really hard to help make the most of what she had. Because she could stand and walk a few steps she could step out of the house and get into my car, so we could take her shopping and have coffee and cake out as a treat.

After 40 days on a hospital ward she has lost all mobility and any muscles she did have are gone. She can't even sit in a chair properly. The hospital did absolutely nothing to maintain my mother's mobility or enable her to return home. They were only focussed on any medical anomaly they could find, but failed catastrophically to assist my mother with anything that she actually wanted or needed. As her mobility declined their response was to mobilise her even less, allow extended periods in bed, provide a reclining chair and use a hoist. At no point did anyone stop and think about treating the things that mattered to maintain the quality of her life. She spent what is most likely her last Christmas on a ward of an acute hospital wondering what day of the week it was and why she was there. It is shocking but sadly very predictable.

As a footnote to this, I grew up next to the UHW [University Hospital of Wales] and watched it being built. My mother was a senior nurse there and before she retired she was director of nursing at a local oncology hospital. She deserved better.

This is another example of "organisational capture" and marks a failure of responsibility leading to a failure to provide appropriate personal care or to link care together across organisational and sector boundaries.

BUILDING RELATIONSHIPS

Relationships between individuals, teams, organisations and stakeholders are key to the transformation that this *paradigm evolution* implies. Work on analysing relationships by the Relationship Foundation for example [12] has informed recent CQC work [13] in twenty local areas. The key concepts of relational value and relational proximity are important to our consideration of mutuality.

KEY CONCEPTS: RELATIONAL VALUE AND RELATIONAL PROXIMITY

The relational audit scorecard is based on two conceptual frameworks for assessing the health of relationships: relational value and relational proximity. They describe the attributes of effective relationships.

Relational value is described by the Whole Systems Partnership and Relationship Foundation as the following:

- Exists between individuals, groups or organisations that can be given a value that is distinct from, though dependent on, the parties to the relationship. For example, the level of *trust* in a relationship can be measured and is distinct from, though dependent on, the level of trustworthiness of the parties to the relationship.
- Has a purpose, or an expected outcome, in a particular context, in other words a relationship is "for something" and can therefore be described as "doing work" toward a specific goal or set of goals. Relational value is something that sets direction.

Relational value is understood to have five attributes:

- *Integrity*: The extent to which there is consistency and cohesiveness between parties.
- *Respect*: The extent to which people treat each other with respect.
- *Fairness*: The extent to which people have equitable shares in the relationship.
- *Empathy*: The extent to which the parties in the relationship have compassion for each other and demonstrate an understanding of each other's needs.
- *Trust*: The extent to which people feel they can rely on others in the relationship.

These attributes of relational value are applied using a sociotechnical framework with six dimensions:

- *Culture*: Including norms and rules; relations between agencies (including shared history); mindsets and worldviews.
- *Vision*: Including ideas about what the future could look like, and expressed goals.
- *People*: Including individual staff skills, development and involvement.
- *Process*: Including routines, standards, briefings, handovers, and working patterns.
- *Infrastructure*: Including the physical space, such as transport and buildings.
- *Technology*: Including the virtual space, such as IT, access to relevant information sources and technological communication.

Relational proximity is a different but related concept that is more focussed on the "closeness" of relationships and aspects that can cause barriers to that. It has five domains:

- *Directness*: How well people communicate in the relationship.
- *Continuity*: The extent to which relationships are consistent over time.
- *Multiplicity*: How well people in the relationship understand each other.
- *Commonality*: The extent to which there are shared aims or goals between parties in a relationship.
- *Parity*: The extent to which there are equitable power relations between people in a relationship.

The key findings concern the importance of investing time and energy in developing strong relationships despite the difficulties involved. The messages about relationships between health and social care staff along with people and organisations from the voluntary sector will be important.

PERSONAL RESPONSIBILITY

This new paradigm of mutuality emphasises the importance of personal responsibility – individual citizens accepting greater responsibility for their own health but in addition the responsibility of clinical staff for people consulting them requires re-emphasising. In the past people registered with their general practitioner, who had overall responsibility for their care, except when that care was transferred, by referral, to a hospital consultant. In the current NHS, with a whole range of autonomous clinicians (salaried and locum GPs, nurse practitioners, clinical pharmacists, counsellors, etc.), responsibility has become more of a group/team or organisation concept. Similarly in the acute hospital, consultants are no longer as "personally" responsible as they used to be – they consult rather than direct – and again it is the team and organisation which is responsible. It seems to me that the concepts of mutual responsibility and mutual dependency are very much part of mutuality and form part of the foundation of this paradigm.

PERSONAL GROUP AND ORGANISATIONAL MATURITY

In addition, I have mentioned maturity before (Chapter 5), but it is another foundation of the mutuality paradigm I am describing. Physical, emotional and psychological maturity are not binary concepts; we all mature as individuals at varying rates and to varying extents. But being able to consider objectively our own health and well-being, being able to make decisions for ourselves, and being able to understand and evaluate evidence and information are key parts of this.

Vignette 5

I met Bernard Brett in 1972 when, as a young student, I helped to convert a barn to an arts centre in Essex. Bernard had cerebral palsy and was physically very disabled, but is now remembered fondly by a sheltered housing scheme named after him in Colchester. He was an early user of a possum keyboard to aid communication and through this grew well beyond the confines of his physical disabilities to study at university level, to lead national work in the field of disability and to inspire all he met with his breadth of insight.

Bernard was the first person I met – and there have been others since – who helped me understand that maturity could be the outcome from bad experience. Bernard's was a birth defect, and I have seen this in a twelve-year-old patient dying with cystic fibrosis. But it is also a feature of some individuals who have overcome addiction, been the victim of domestic violence or abuse, or been forced to migrate from their homeland. Many are damaged by these experiences; some learn from them and it is that learning which we need to celebrate, as it provides the maturity I am talking about. Of course, maturity is not a binary concept – it is a spectrum and in the context of empowerment to take responsibility in the primary care sector we will need to give the process time to develop. But just like the analogy with secondary education discussed in Chapter 7 where all young people are exposed to the same education system and expected to behave maturely in terms of school rules, exam performance and personal development, so we need to empower people in the primary care sector to have responsibility for their lives. Of course, this maturity does not only apply to us as individuals; team and organisations also mature and need to act maturely if they are to be successful.

GOVERNANCE

Finally, the mutuality paradigm is dependent on sound governance – just as all organisations and sectors of activity are. It will be apparent from earlier chapters that I believe sound governance has not been assured in the primary care sector in the past (see Chapter 3 for example) due to design issues in the sector affecting the balance between power, responsibility and trust in both organisational governance and clinical governance [14]. Through transformation of governing arrangements within the primary care sector and ensuring it becomes fit for purpose in the digital world that we are moving into, it requires a safe framework to ensure that it is safe for citizens to trust the sector, safe for staff to trust their careers to the sector, and safe for the wider community to trust the sector with its responsibilities for use of resources and provision of care. In order to meet this agenda, I feel the following aspects need reflecting on:

1. The extent to which provider organisations are open to challenge and scrutiny. Public sector bodies are required to publish their accounts and face challenges about them, from non-executive directors as well as the public in meetings "held in public". Existing arrangements for professional partnerships are much less rigorous – no published accounts, no public accountability and no real challenge from commissioners or other stakeholders.

2. The extent to which individuals working in the sector should have clinical autonomy. The freedom to act independently or be required to work as part of teams, accepting responsibility to and management by, the team.
3. The role local citizen's play in the arrangements governing the organisation. How powerful is their voice in directing the organisation?

REFERENCES

1. Langdon J. 2018. Tessa Jowell obituary: the 'people politician'. *Guardian*, May 13. https://www.theguardian.com/politics/2018/may/13/the-people-politician-tessa-jowell-obituary.
2. Richards T. 2017. The response to the "cancer drugs scandal" must fully involve patients – An essay by Tessa Richards. *BMJ* 359:j4956.
3. Kempis TA. 1994. *The Imitation of Christ*. http://www.catholicplanet.com/ebooks/Imitation-of-Christ.pdf.
4. Starey N. 1996. The primary care trust: Coordination for cohesion. In G Meads (ed), *Future Options for General Practice*. Radcliffe Medical, Oxford.
5. Care Quality Commission. 2015. Inclusion Healthcare Social Enterprise CIC: Overview and CQC inspections. https://www.cqc.org.uk/location/1-572021031.
6. General Medical Council. 2013. Good medical practice. GMC, Manchester. https://www.gmc-uk.org/ethical-guidance/ethical-guidance-for-doctors/good-medical-practice.
7. West M. 2016. What can you achieve through better team working in an organisation? Affina Organisation Development, October 4. https://www.affinaod.com/article/can-achieve-better-team-working-organisation.
8. Care Quality Commission. 2017. *The State of Care in General Practice 2014–2017*. CQC, London.
9. Care Quality Commission. 2018. *Beyond Barriers*. CQC, London.
10. Commission on the Future of Health and Social Care in England. 2015. https://www.kingsfund.org.uk/projects/commission-future-health-and-social-care-england.
11. Gowlad B. 2017, May 22. Episode 64: Helen Parker – General practice lessons from New Zealand – Part 1 [podcast]. https://ockham.healthcare/episode-64-helen-parker-general-practice-lessons-from-new-zealand-part-1/.
12. Relationship Foundation. 2016. https://www.amazon.co.uk/Relational-Lens-Understanding-Stakeholder-Relationships/dp/1107155762/ref=sr_1_1?s=books&ie=UTF8&qid=1507908233&sr=1-1&keywords=the+relational+lens.
13. Care Quality Commission. 2018. Beyond barriers: How older people move between health and social care in England. Annex: Relational audit – Summary of findings. https://www.cqc.org.uk/sites/default/files/20180702_beyond-barriers_annex_relational-audit-summary-findings.pdf.
14. Sparrow N. 2017, August 10. Nigel's surgery 64: Effective governance arrangements in GP practices. www.cqc.org.uk/guidance-providers/gps/nigels-surgery-64-effective-governance-arrangements-gp-practices.

9

Thinking outside the box

HERCULES' FIFTH LABOUR: THE AUGEAN STABLES

Unlike earlier labours which were based on physical strength, cleaning the stables of King Augeas required Hercules to think outside the box; by diverting a river he cleared the mountain of dung. We have to believe that what looks impossible can be achieved if you look at it differently – from outside the box. In this case I will be using elements from systems theory (see previous chapters) to analyse the dynamics of the system while not being constrained by structure (anatomy), history or perceived wisdom.

As the digital revolution infiltrates all aspects of modern life, so the implications for health and welfare services have to come under scrutiny. We can describe a coherent vision for the future of the primary care sector within a national welfare system: one that inspires everyone involved; supports their ongoing commitment to the sector; and meets the needs of the community as part of one seamless system which also includes the specialist healthcare and residential social care sectors.

Just as the industrial revolution of the eighteenth and nineteenth centuries, the social and technological revolutions of the twentieth century have each evolved or rolled on from each other, and innovators have, in their turn, climbed on the shoulders of pioneers. So all aspects of the digital revolution also have their roots in history and again we stand on the shoulders of the pioneers who have driven the National Health Service (NHS) through its first seventy years and their predecessors who developed the welfare system in earlier generations – their heritage is our legacy and it is that heritage – NHS Mk 1 which provides the prepared ground for NHS Mk 2 – it includes:

- Being based on a *social contract* where universal coverage is funded by general taxation and care is largely free at the point of need.
- Central government funding of the system, but this has involved facing the same issues of the gap between demand and available resources as every other developed health economy. These include rising costs as health technologies have become more expensive and rising demand as the population's rising

life expectancy and appetite for healthcare have increased. Although many in the population say they may be prepared to pay more for their NHS [1], the taxpayer has also to be increasingly aware that the NHS model may become unsustainable. When the NHS budget grows like Topsy, it threatens to starve other sectors of the resources they deserve in order to meet the other needs of the population for education, defence, prisons and pensions, for example. Recent years of austerity in the economy have magnified this effect, as differential cuts to government spending have sought to protect health and social care spending. However, the roots of the economic challenges of the last decade run deeper. There is a global shortage of capital in the West, as the needs of emerging economies in countries like China and India require attention, along with a failure to plan for sustainable development in the UK welfare sector and a failure to appreciate the implications of demographic social and technological forces. As a result the NHS and social care sectors have been squeezed and the pips have been squeaking. Calls for a special NHS tax, "hypothecated" or not [2], is not the point. The issues remain and cannot be addressed simply by more sticking plaster. The inverse care law [3] becomes inflated in these circumstances: the strong promote their interest at the expense of the weak and those with greatest health needs such as the frail elderly and children at risk lose out to those who shout loudest for rapid access and priority attention. The NHS labour shortage sucks in scarce resources from around the world in a way that is as unsustainable as it is unfair.

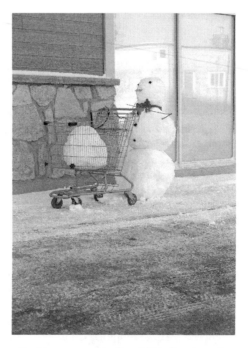

Pushing a snowball uphill is hard work.

IMPLICATIONS

- We have to recognise that the Care Quality Commission's (CQC) methodology sometimes penalises those who seek to reverse this by its focus on accessibility and patient survey results rather than focussing on the extent to which the organisation is meeting the needs of the most vulnerable and challenging the inverse care law [3].
- Being a service rather than a system – like the fire service or the ambulance or police services – designed to meet the needs of the population. In the early years, each service was administered and overseen by committees. Then in the 1960s, there was a general management revolution designed to increase efficiency and effectiveness [4] but always in an uncomfortable bed with the clinical tribes of the medical and nursing professionals, whose power general managers struggled to harness. This was also a service lacking cohesion, with no one coherent hierarchy like an army or the police force – where hospital and home are different worlds, while social care needs were largely met within the family or local community. Nevertheless, it remained a service rather than a system serving the community, uniform across the kingdom, regimented and hierarchical, in command and control mode – not an integrated system like the Swiss railway or the stock exchange – focussing on quality and safety, while the NHS focusses on efficiency and bureaucracy (see Chapter 3 for a fuller discussion).
- This history has to call into question whether government can any longer realistically deliver on its key functions: to ensure the safety and security of the country as well as sustaining the welfare system. This may risk the NHS withering on the vine as it struggles to adapt and thrive in a new world which it was not designed for, and with its resources at the mercy of short-term political cycles.
  - In the early years the NHS struggled for resources in a world of food and fuel rationing (a world of reusing bandages) where social cohesion was built on victory in World War II and elements of communitarianism (from meals on wheels to union power). A world where families were strong and provided mutual support, queuing was inevitable and you gave up your seat to the elderly and held the door open for a woman.
  - In the current environment where the death of "community" has proven premature, neoliberalism is regarded as a swamp to be drained, global warming is labelled "fake news" and albatrosses feed their young on regurgitated plastic. It would seem that any government must respect the population's views. If it is to be electable it must work with the grain of its electorate's culture and accept that this means redefining its *social contract* to ensure welfare provision for the whole population (based on individual need) funded through central taxation and delivered through a system which is designed for the digital world.
    - A world which has left behind historic libertarian and egalitarian as the sole dimensions of political thinking.
    - Aspires to accept the reality of green life – sustainable development and a heritage of hope for our children.

- Rejects the narrow negativism of populism, while acknowledging the failures of neoliberalism.
- This is a culture where "Brexit" or "remain" arguments are sterile, and health economics is an analytical and decision support tool rather than a determinant of health policy. This is a world where the welfare system is designed to support every citizen throughout their life, to promote their independence and autonomy, to protect the weak, to care about the future, and to command the trust and respect of the population, but defined by key design features, that is, open and accountable, confidential, trustworthy and reliable.

In this chapter we will continue our journey by looking at the implications for all those groups, organisations and individuals who are affected by the impact of the digital revolution on the "out-of-hospital" welfare sector.

- We will consider how professional roles, responsibilities, relationships values and behaviours might adapt.
- We will look at the organisations involved in the sector and how fit they are for the roles and responsibilities they face.
- We will look at some aspects of relationships – both those within the primary care sector and those between the sector and the wider world – and how they are evolving because that will underpin and ensure safety and quality assurance in the new world.

PROFESSIONS

Power within NHS Mk 1 was largely in the hands of the members of the medical, nursing and allied professions. They had earned the confidence of the public, were trusted and respected, had often joined their professions from a sense of vocation (see Chapter 8), worked hard, and enjoyed a privileged social position somehow outside the class system that still underpins British society.

But society and the social context within which the professions live has changed dramatically since 1946, and these changes have profound implications to the professions and their members, sometimes challenging their cultural norms and identities.

In 2017, I took a few weeks to walk the South West Coast Path – 630 miles of opportunity to reflect, to talk to people along the way and to put in place some my own experiences as a family doctor since the 1970s. The opportunity and time to reflect, while undisturbed by modern technology, has been influential in the analysis underpinning this book. But particularly in this section where, rather than describing the structure, functions and behaviour of professions, I shall share some reflections on the forces operating on the professional workforce and their consequences.

1. The medical professions have served society for hundreds of years, but as Illich [5] pointed out they may be bad for health, just as teachers may damage learning and the clergy be a barrier to spiritual growth. Unless the members

of the professions can redefine their purpose and culture, they risk losing their place in society. The implications are as great for dentists and pharmacists as they are for doctors and nurses; all the caring provider professions have to adapt to the needs of a modern digital world or become stranded on the shores of a new world where professional values become corporate, allegiance is to the manager of the service rather than to the patient, and the professional body of knowledge has to be based on experience rather than data and facts that anyone can read online.

2. We live in a "post-family" society where population migration and loneliness go hand in hand – where single parenting, intergenerational tensions over wealth sharing, and a weakening of the commitment of the young to care for the old are moulding the way the medical and nursing professions are working. I have seen the stress felt by carers of a terminally ill man by his distant family wanting him to be cared for at home and to be a part of the team making that happen, but the local care team struggling to cope. I have also seen the catastrophic effects of dementia on a family and the inequity of family wealth – where an old man on a good pension can be well supported in his own home while his children and grandchildren struggle to put fuel in their cars to visit him. As a family doctor, I confront these stressors every day and I am not sure it is my role to balance them, but I do see how these tensions are eroding social cohesion.

3. We live in a world of instant access to news, to data and to services (banking, shopping and entertainment are just three examples). They should help us to understand why the population we serve as healthcare professionals requires similar access to welfare services; the culture of queuing for the bus, rationing and waiting for a council house has been consigned to history. Consumers want to buy strawberries in January, want to watch a TV programme when it suits them and have instant access to healthcare. In this world, NHS Mk 1 can never be good enough; no matter how much extra money is put in, the model can never deliver. You can keep updating a Morris Minor, but it will never meet the needs of the modern driver or passenger – and NHS Mk 1 cannot cope in the digital instant-access world – sticking plaster simply covers up the underlying problems.

4. The talent pool fuelling recruitment to the nursing and medical professions has changed. Nursing has moved to become a more academic profession with nurses studying for degrees rather than following a largely apprenticeship-based training to registration. We have never trained enough nurses and always relied on migration to make up the shortfall. This approach is no longer acceptable. We have to accept that it sucks in talent at the expense of weakening donor countries and their healthcare systems, and should never be more than a short-term sticking plaster fix of a workforce gap. Our workforce plans should also recognise:

- The short length of the average nurse's career and the transferability of their skills to better paid jobs.
- The medical profession is becoming increasingly feminised and, as in the rest of society, part-time (as compared to the seven-day commitment of my father's time at the start of the NHS, and the one-in-two rotas of my training and the 24/7 contract when I joined the GP performers list in the 1980s).

* The transformation caused by the European Working Time Directive, the GP contract changes of 1998, and more importantly the social trend to shorter working hours and a life focussed on leisure as a replacement for vocation and the drudgery of the wage-slave years.

The result is an expectation that a full-time GP partner may do six clinical sessions each week and only a minority will do extra out-of-hours work. The difficulty recruiting to the medical and nursing professions is due to the mismatch between these issues: we can't recruit to the old model and the current position has not been matched by a model that both meets the needs of the population and is attractive to potential recruits. We need a vision for the future of the service, for the future of the professionals committing their future to the sector and of what professionalism means in the digital world. We also need a new "sector" model which can restore confidence among the workforce, the people who need them and commissioners. This I shall describe in the following chapter, but not before considering the other factors which the model has to address.

PROFESSIONALISM

1. Universal access to the internet means that the *body of knowledge* held by members of a profession is no longer sacrosanct – the power this knowledge gave members is diluted and just as we can all be armchair historians, knowledgeable sportsman and do our own tax forms so everyone can google their symptoms, look at the evidence about best treatment, and read about the wonders of genetic healthcare or cancer diagnosis. The reality is that if knowledge is power, then in the NHS Mk 2 much of that power has moved. But knowledge is not everything, and when people are emotionally involved, worried or unwell, they still need support and advice to interpret the data and to balance their decision making by looking holistically at the issues they face, and to have confidence that the advice they base their decision on is less biased than that coming online through a multinational, corporate, impersonal website or source. This points towards the future of professionalism in the out-of-hospital sector and beyond.

2. While direct provision of care – assessing, diagnosing, organising and coordinating treatment and ensuring sufficient continuity of care to ensure confidence and assure quality – will remain important, can we really support "professional capture" by the holding of our lifelong biographical record, trapped in the GP's surgery? Even though it is on SystmOne or EMIS rather than in a Lloyd George envelope? In this digital world the record has to become *ours* – it is our story, from our birth and baby tests to our deaths in all its messy detail. In addition this "biographical" record has to support and inform our "episodic care" in hospital and the wider primary care sector as well as care when we travel the world – whenever and wherever we need help. To be clear – professionalism requires that our individual biography's transfer to become our own responsibility and are available to inform our care at all times.

Vignette 1

I vividly remember an American gentleman consulting me in the 1990s. He had been ill while holidaying in Thailand and was on his way back home. He wanted further tests and medicines while in the UK and had all his health biography "on file", including his MRI scan from Thailand. For me this was liberating. We could have an informed consultation, and I know he found the consultation and his brief experience of the UK health service beneficial. It was a chance to review and discuss his problems informed by his results and a chance to answer his questions about what it all meant.

* All of us should hold our own record, and everyone we consult, whether online or in person, should add to it and use it – with our consent. It would be an unfair and an exaggerated comparison to compare it to the mediaeval restriction of literacy and education among the general population by professionalising its distribution through monasteries and their monks – really an abuse of professionalism – but it is not *that* unfair a comparison.
* In the world I sketch here and in the final chapter, the "New NHS Mk 2" service becomes centred around us, every individual citizen, the users, rather than on those providing the service, i.e. the professional carers and their organisations.
* CQC has been looking at digital providers in recent months – the lack of reliable links between online providers and the rest of the NHS and local health economies raises a concern when access to medicines, tests and advice is not informed by, and does not inform their biographical record. Nevertheless the convenience and instant access the digital providers offer requires that NHS Mk 2 develops a "digital" offer to the whole population.

The role of the professions, the core values and purpose of professionalism has to evolve to focus more on interpretation, support, trust and understanding – to holding our hand through the pathway of our pathology, to guiding us through the decisions we face as our life transitions and to hear our distress in ways that the digital platforms are deaf to. There is more to being a family doctor or community nurse now and in NHS Mk 2 than can be delivered online or in a walk-in centre. What we have to design is a system which provides for us, both for when we need digital, instant access and for when we need our hands held. Our biographical record has to be our "golden thread" linking and informing our care no matter where our journey takes us. And it has to be "Ours". The GMC guidance to doctors "Good Medical Practice" [6] requires review to ensure that the golden thread retains its credibility and reliability and supports healthcare delivery. If citizens own and appreciate the importance of the golden thread "Our medical record", then they are much more likely to agree to all their data being included in it.

3. Professional relationships are constrained by their history and will reflect NHS Mk 1 design for many years. The relationship between the care providing professions and people they care for also fails to reflect accurately the new balance of power that the digital revolution has ushered in. As with many national services, relationships between doctors, nurses and the other professional groups involved in care provision are well demarcated by culture – from separate parking spaces to uniforms – with clear definition of roles, responsibilities and authorities. But recent times have seen a trend to skill substitution to multi-professional education and to team working. In NHS Mk 2, the community will still need the same skills and expertise to be available to help meet their needs, but the teams providing care will need to be designed to be fit for purpose – shared objectives, common records and coherent care plans, available 24/7 and with greater clarity about power, responsibility and accountability for performance. Similarly, the relationships between individuals and their carers have altered since the days of Balint [7] when the relationship was the key therapeutic instrument. For many people, empowerment to take responsibility of their own health remains rhetoric rather than reality. In the digital world this is changing; people are accessing healthcare online when it suits them, unconstrained by the historic design of NHS Mk 1. In inspecting the digital sector, CQC has been challenged to define best practice among both treatment and consultation providers, both in terms of the quality and safety of the services and in the relationship they have with people using the service. In addition, the rules of engagement between digital providers and other parts of the health economy are sometimes not close enough, such that the holder of the biographical patient record (currently the GP) may not be informed about treatment provided from a digital provider, including occasions where the risk of harm is real rather than theoretical. In NHS Mk 2 the risk of care fragmentation driven by fragmented records is too great and must be designed out of the system.

4. Modern technology has supported the transfer of more care from hospital to home, for example day-case surgery and early discharge, systematic care for those with diabetes and COPD in general practice, home dialysis, and outreach specialist teams for people with multiple sclerosis or cancer. But unless the parties redefine their roles in the care journeys involved, care quality cannot be assured. When specialist nurses report to their acute trust employers, community nurses to the community trust, and care package providers to social services, we should not be surprised if care is compromised by competing priorities and tribal perspectives. Professionalism among all of those providing home-based care has to mean commitment to meeting the needs of the individuals they are supporting. This implies and requires:

   • Team, as well as individual, appraisal and performance management arrangements (as described in earlier chapters); aligned individual and team objectives; clear communication arrangements; and lines of accountability for performance.

   • Aggregation of the fragmented accidents of history. Small general practices, walk-in centres and hubs, dentists and opticians, community nurses, occupational therapists, physiotherapists, social workers, health visitors and the population they care for have to commit to becoming part of one team, one organisation and one point of access. This moves beyond current recommendations [8] but nevertheless this and the *Five Year Forward* Vanguard projects such as Encompass in Kent have illustrated the potential of aggregation and NHS Mk 2 needs to be radical if it is to move beyond strategic intentions and papers which have littered bins for too long. Current arrangements for urgent and emergency care at home also need to become part of this. GP out-of-hours services, NHS 111, ambulance and paramedic services, minor injury units and walk-in centres currently work in relative isolation – a situation which is confusing to everyone – and nobody really believes that efficient and effective care is possible in this fragmented world where the lack of access to the biographical record when it is most needed should be a matter of shame to the whole service.

Vignette 2

Molly, aged fifty-eight, has multiple sclerosis (MS) and breast cancer. She is supported at home by the specialist MS nursing team, the hospice care team, a social services care package, her family, and occasional input from the GP team and community nursing staff. All was running smoothly until the flu arrived one weekend – and the out-of-hours services had to step in.

COORDINATION

- Reformation of the current contracting and commissioning arrangements for home-based care. CQC has found a huge amount of really good care in its inspection reports in the primary care sector, but when "long-term conditions" exclude those born with congenital and genetic conditions, those with deafness and blindness, those with multiple sclerosis and those with psoriasis then the "good" in CQC reports has to be qualified to "good for LTC covered by the contract". Similarly, when issues such as dementia, addiction, cancer care and smoking cessation are ignored by providers, it is the absence of any sensitive local commissioning that is the root cause, for current arrangements fail to address the reality of the health needs of the population and the people who make it up. *General medical services (GMS)/personal medical services (PMS) and alternative provider medical services (APMS) contracts are not appropriate vehicles for ensuring the people receive the quality of care they deserve.*
- It is also widely acknowledged that specialist care in hospital – from accident and emergency (A&E) to intensive therapy unit (ITU), from ward to outpatients – can gain much from effective community links, not just around discharging the frail elderly filling their beds, but also from ensuring that the hospital can provide the range of specialist care that the population needs. Reformation of the home-based care sector has to include a commitment to

dismantling the "Berlin Wall" between hospital-based care and home-based care. Local people flood to A&E, fill the hospital's beds and their outpatient clinics. With coordination and care plans designed around individual patients needs, could come better joined-up care. This could mean diabetic services integrating hospital and home-based care, cancer multidisciplinary team (MDT) meetings opening up to welcome and consider the patient's perspective [9], perhaps through engaging with the patient's GP as their advocate and care coordinator. Even using Skype to shrink the gap could work. Similarly, considering emergency care across the home and hospital makes sense, as does care in almost every department of the hospital. In the digital world, specialist services have to meet the needs of the population rather than expect patients to remain supplicant and subservient to the needs of the hospital.

FORM FOR FUNCTION

In approaching the clearance of the Augean stables task, Hercules might as a GP partnership have referred the task to the hospital as "beyond our experience", as a satellite site for a corporate provider the task would be referred for central guidance, a community nursing team/trust would have ordered a large number of incontinence pads, and an optical provider would have wanted more lenses. All would see the task from their perspective, and the river would not have been diverted.

- In the current NHS Mk 1, the out-of-hospital or home-based sector has evolved over the last seventy years to address the needs of the population for general medical, general dental, pharmaceutical, optical, community nursing and social care. Care has been provided holistically to the whole population, throughout their lives, and needs have either been met within the sector or by a process of referral for specialist treatment. Coordination between the various small providers in any location is not encouraged by the framework of contracting mechanisms that has resourced the sector, so people often have to visit several providers for treatment. A simple water infection or earache might involve an out-of-hours provider appointment, a GP appointment, a visit to a local pharmacy, a hearing test at the optician's and a referral to hospital for a scan, for example. All this involves transport, time off work or school, multiple history taking, examinations, and records – hugely inefficient, frustrating for everyone involved, and expensive.
- There have been many projects, pilots and schemes aimed at improving coordination within the sector, and between it and the specialist and social care sectors. But from the days of GP fundholding to the primary care home and Vanguard models and the new accountable care systems and GP networks, they have all sought to improve the efficiency and effectiveness of care in the sector without redesigning considering the organisational form issues – from the self-employed GP partnership model to the private optician chain and the NHS trust community nursing provider and the local authority social care system.
- In the NHS Mk 2 "digital welfare" sector where the Augean stables need cleaning, the *functions* of the home-based care sector deserve reconsideration

and the *form* or organisational design needs to be rethought to become fit for purpose. We cannot carry on with the Morris Minor and simply retrofit an electric motor and modern audio/info console. This method of evolutionary development of the primary care sector has lasted seventy years. It is admired around the world [10], trusted by and large, popular with the population, rated by CQC at over eighty percent "good" – the best-performing sector of all rated sectors in the world. But it is not designed to meet the needs of the population. The functions that the sector is now needing to respond to include:

- Online consulting and medicine supply seven days a week and twenty-four hours a day.
- Complex care needs for the frail elderly with multiple co-morbidities, at home or in the nursing and residential care sector.
- The demand for care whenever and wherever the people want it.
- Care after rapid discharge from specialist treatment – day-case hysterectomy, cholecystectomy, outpatient chemotherapy and endoscopy for example.
- Specialist nursing care at home – for people with cancer, multiple sclerosis and learning disabilities for example.
- Complex dental procedures – such as dental implants being provided in the community.
- Home-based care of macular degeneration and venous ulcers, deep vein thrombosis and diabetes.
- Rapid access to specialist opinion and treatment when required.

But the uncomfortable truth remains that the current design of the sector has also fallen short in introducing evidence-based best practice when it challenges commercial interests. For example the percentage of babies who are breastfed remains stubbornly as low as when I qualified and this is a scandal because it is bad for babies health [12]. The public's need for effective measures to address issues such as alcohol dependency, substance misuse and obesity are not adequately responded to; and the need for focussing on issues of loneliness, adolescent mental, distress and the systems through which children and the vulnerable are safeguarded are only a few examples of many issues where the current arrangements fall short. Our attention is grabbed by the day's news, and the outstanding examples of exceptional care in these and other areas are not learned from, because the sector is not *designed* to learn. The sector does not work as a system; it remains a service. The primary care sector perpetuates and persists within the paradigm of the medical model through system archetypes which are characterised by *supply-induced demand, boom and bust, and tragedy of the commons rather than shifting the burden or escalation where adapting and learning are fundamental. NHS Mk 1 has become trapped in a way of thinking which leads to vicious cycles rather than virtuous ones.*

To move beyond these archetypes and paradigms, the sector's mental models and mindsets demand review. If the stables are to be drained and the functions delivered, we need to design a system that can think differently – outside the box "by design".

There has been a mantra in recent years that the only answer to the problems of the sector – from workforce shortages to rising demand, to CQC inadequate ratings to ambulances and trolleys queuing outside emergency departments – is "We need more resources" (i.e. an extra X billion pounds for the NHS, a greater percent of the cake for primary care, more GPs and more nurses). Now it may well be that a "fit for purpose" sector will require additional cash and people to deliver on its functions, but at least there should be the opportunity to focus on the agreed functions and assess the sector's efficiency. Let us start by designing a system fit for the functions which we, the individuals making up the population, require it to fulfil. Let us agree on the form which supports the delivery of these functions and only then consider the resources required to power the system – human, community, volunteers and professionals as well as cash.

RELATIONSHIPS

The essence of my previous book, *The Challenge for Primary Care* [11], was that the sector needed to demonstrate its trustworthiness if it was to thrive. In the new digital NHS Mk 2, the essence is that it is only through strong, therapeutic and supportive relationships between individuals, teams and organisations in the sectors making up NHS Mk 2, that we can design and deliver a sector that can be trusted with the public's confidence and cash.

At the centre of this is the relationship between the user of the service (someone we sometimes call the patient) or the individual citizen and the organisation providing that service. In the digital world, as already discussed in earlier sections, the user that the NHS Mk 1 service was designed for has matured. Today's user is better educated, has instant access to all the resources of the internet, is more leisured and more isolated, and less compliant and less supplicant. To establish and maintain successful therapeutic and supportive relationships in this world still requires the commitment of both sides, a continuity of responsibility, reliable comprehensive records, a respect for confidentiality and a respect for each other. Since the days of Balint [7], the value of this relationship to promoting individuals' health and well-being has been paramount, has been a key feature in many CQC "outstanding" ratings, and shines through the feedback on NHS choices. But we have designed a service which promotes instant access over continuity of care, delegation and skill substitution to provide more efficient care, and has turned many clinicians into guideline and template slaves rather than trusted advocates. Changes to the way the NHS contracts for general dental services have also changed relationships in the sector, and the state of the nation's teeth remains suboptimal, with access to care an accident of geography, too many people suffering with dental pain presenting to emergency and out-of-hours medical services, and too many children requiring dental extractions in hospital.

In the social care sector, the relationship between client, carer and social services remains problematic rather than constructive. Past experience, heavy caseload, staff inexperience and funding streams all contribute to this, but they act as barriers to all our desires to put the individual – be they a vulnerable child or a frail elderly person – at the centre of planning and care delivery. Having dealt with too many safeguarding concerns, read too many serious case reviews, and questioned both health and social care professionals, it seems to me that sometimes it is the design of our health and social care systems which promotes risk rather than prevents harm.

If the individual citizen's relationship with the sector remains key to the sector's trustworthiness, then so do the relationships within and between the teams and organisations providing care. If Hercules is to clean the stable, he needs a plan which assesses the whole problem he faces and he needs to devise a plan in which all those involved recognise as appropriate, i.e. diverting the river might need heavy lifting gear or machinery and planning permission, disrupt many animals and citizen's lives, and alter the local fisherman's way of life. Similarly, meeting the needs of families with health and social care problems requires coordination and cooperation, team working and effective leadership. Currently, all of these elements seem to have become more difficult to deliver. The end result being too many frail elderly blocking beds in acute hospitals, too many safeguarding referrals to overstretched social service departments, and too many of the most vulnerable (such as those with severe learning disabilities or children with complex needs) being failed.

The relationship between those organisations in the community that provide for the community's welfare, both health and social care, are similarly strong or weak as a result of historic experience rather than any comprehensive, systematic plan to maximise the effective delivery of compassionate, well-coordinated care.

NHS Mk 1 involved GP practices nearly always set up as private sector professional partnerships where the GPs provide the premises, employ the staff, capitalise the business and provide the care for their registered list. They would be in competition with other neighbouring practices, and may have positive or negative relationships with them as a result of experience. Similarly, the relationship between other organisations involved in providing care – dentists, community nursing, community pharmacy, social services, community care providers, nursing and residential care home providers – has been largely informal, with no shared vision of what each is trying to achieve and no agreed programme of cooperation or service development. The emergence of out-of-hours GP cooperatives in the 1990s served to promote a culture of joint working and broke down some barriers. Recent initiatives such as primary care homes, GP federations and networks, and super practices have provided further impetus to improve professional and organisational relationships. Unfortunately, sometimes there are contractual barriers to such developments; the GP contracting frameworks and self-employed independent contractor model can be impediments, for example.

A further dimension to the relationship network underpinning care delivery is that with the community. In its inspection programme the CQC came across examples of strong relationships, with real commitment from both care providers and local communities to ensure they worked well together in the interests of local people. This "communitarian" focus was sometimes rewarded with an "outstanding"

CQC rating when it demonstrated a commitment by the provider to deliver a service designed to support and strengthen the local community, that is working with the voluntary sector, local councils, education and local businesses to ensure the provider was meeting the community's needs "by design", an often virtuous circle of success where recruitment, commitment, satisfaction and rewards follow each other. However, too often the CQC found providers drowning in the demand from local people for access to healthcare, seeing themselves as under siege and unable to provide the level of service they aspired to. Too often this can become a vicious circle of decline where the service fails because there is no alternative. The CQC's special measures programme may provide some short-term support, an APMS contract or a merger may also be tried, but they are really sticking-plaster approaches to more deeply entrenched problems – cleaning the stables requires a different approach.

For NHS Mk 2 out-of-hospital care in the digital world to be sustainable – both for a failing organisation in special measures and for an "outstanding" organisation to thrive – it needs to be driven by a shared vision of their future to which they can commit to and aim for.

REFERENCES

1. Cream J, Maguire G and Robertson R. 2018. How have public attitudes to the NHS changed over the past three decades? https://www.kingsfund.org.uk/publications/how-have-public-attitudes-to-nhs-changed.
2. Hayes A. 2018. Replace national insurance with tax dedicated to NHS and social care, experts say. *Sky News*, February 5. https://news.sky.com/story/replace-national-insurance-with-tax-dedicated-to-nhs-and-social-care-say-experts-11237695.
3. Hart JT. 1971. The inverse care law. *Lancet* 297:405–12. https://www.thelancet.com/journals/lancet/article/PIIS0140-6736(71)92410-X/fulltext.
4. Griffiths R. 1983. NHS management inquiry. *BMJ* 287:1391–4.
5. Illich I. 1975. *Limits to Medicine: Medical Nemesis; The Expropriation of Health*. Penguin, London.
6. General Medical Council. 2013. Good medical practice. GMC, Manchester. https://www.gmc-uk.org/ethical-guidance/ethical-guidance-for-doctors/good-medical-practice.
7. Balint M. 1957. *The Doctor, His Patient and the Illness*. Pitman Medical Press, London.
8. Charles A. 2018. Reimagining community services [blog]. National Voices, February 5. https://www.nationalvoices.org.uk/blogs/reimagining-community-services.
9. Richards T. 2017. The response to the "cancer drugs scandal" must fully involve patients – An essay by Tessa Richards. *BMJ* 359:j4956.
10. Starfield B. 1994. Is primary care essential? *Lancet* 344:1129–33.
11. Starey N. 2003. *The Challenge for Primary Care*. Radcliffe Medical Press, Abingdon.
12. Modi N. 2017. Attitudes of breastfeeding must change in UK. *Guardian*. August 1.8.2017.

10

New dawn: Welfare in NHS Mk 2 – A new social compact

INTRODUCTION

It is the nature of describing any vision of the future that there is an inevitable uncertainty of detail, the possibility that events and developments along the way will distort the vision, but nevertheless a description matters. It matters because otherwise the heritage of those we climb on the shoulders of is at risk. In the emerging digital world around the primary care sector there is a toxic mix of role uncertainty, organisational and pathway confusion, a rising tide of complex need, and sometimes inappropriate demand. The toxic mix which is being threatened by austerity in the specialist and social care sectors, leading to unresourced workload transfering into the primary care sector, staffing problems, partly, as a result of our Brexit leaving the European Union, and a declining share of the National Health Service (NHS) resource cake (no matter the kind words of NHS England, any extra cash has been sucked up to balance the books in the specialist sector, as it has been throughout the seventy years of NHS Mk 1, while the out-of-hospital sector's share declines towards seven percent of the total NHS cake). In this environment, detailing a vision around which the sector can emerge with renewed vigour; a vision to inspire clinicians to commit with their careers and energy primary care to a vision describing a system which the people across the country can trust and rely on to provide high-quality, coordinated, safe care. This might be considered tricky and brave, but I consider it only makes the task more pressing. So, this vision is a *direction of travel* – a template to be tested and a system to be explored. Its feedback loops, its catalysts and its risks need to be detailed and then explored over time so that the vision can inspire and grow as it evolves. Our own future health and welfare are both the prize of success and at risk if the scope of our vision is too narrow and our mindset is too negative.

- Our journey through the history and physiology of the current primary care sector in the NHS is now complete (Chapters 1–8). Its analysis of the various factors and forces contributing to the dichotomy that is the current "out-of-hospital" welfare system gives us a perspective from which to describe what the future system will look like. The dichotomy is between the findings of the Care Quality Commission (CQC) inspection programmes in the segments of the sector – over eighty percent "good" in English general practice – but in a sector where workforce crises, poor morale and distress provide daily headlines; where fiscal austerity meets rising demand from the complex co-morbidities of the frail elderly; where the squeezed needs of the vulnerable whose alternative avenues have been closed; all of which squeeze the bottom line in organisations whose share of the NHS cake has fallen to less than eight percent.

- Our journey has now equipped us with the brush to paint a very different picture of what "NHS Mk 2" or the "national welfare system" might look like in future years. This ought to be a system designed to meet the needs of people in the digital world – a world where the country remains committed to providing welfare services for all who need them, free at the point of need, paid for through central taxation, providing all the services for people living either at home or in the nursing and care home sector – in the community, and with access to specialist services when necessary (some in a residential "hospital" building and some others through outreach specialist services provided to people living in the community). A world where people have been freed from the tyranny of lifelong servitude, have greater independence and more opportunity to dream their dreams, but also a world of greater loneliness and anxiety, where the burden of frailty and vulnerability pose new risks to our quality of life, and the desire we all have to provide hope and opportunity for our children, our legacy for future generations.

- So this chapter paints a picture – one of many possible variants, one designed to climb on the shoulders of our heritage, to recognise the experience of innovators and to add new fuel to the fire which, as CQC inspections have found, still burns strongly in those providing care and in the communities they serve. The key brushstrokes outlining this picture are

  - Responsible citizenship
  - Redefined professionalism
  - Mutuality
  - Organisational integration

  They have been described earlier in the book along with their derivation. They are needed to enable form and function to offer synergy in place of dissonance, virtuous cycles instead of vicious ones, and hope in place of despair.

- Supported to deliver on its *functions* by a clarity and redefinition of what the sector can and cannot provide, what the individual citizen can and cannot expect from the welfare system or from the wider community and what they need to provide for themselves or take out insurance against.

- The *form* or forms in this system will need to be designed to deliver the agreed functions, to inspire confidence and to be sufficiently malleable to evolve to meet the needs of the community. The system should balance rights with responsibilities, respect confidence and value trustworthy relationships, and whose systems and processes are open to scrutiny, and where individuals are accountable for their performance. In moving toward providing primary welfare services "at scale", i.e. through larger organisations with the capacity and capability to safely deliver the functions and lead the delivery of high quality care, we have to ensure that they do not become so distant as to threaten the provision of *personal* care – that would threaten the sector's heritage. The relationship between individual citizens and their personal, professional advisers remains as important as ever, but does it always need to necessitate a face-to-face consultation with a named GP to legitimise it? Or might this constrain relationships too much? Could "virtual" contact replace face to face? Should other clinicians supplement the GP in providing such personal care and support?

- This system is resourced, or *fuelled*, as much by individual and community commitment as it is by cash, and it rewards and celebrates excellence and commitment, just as an electric car harvests energy when it brakes and recycled compost reinvigorates our gardens. This then is a green world where fossil fuel is valued as heritage and the NHS Mk 2 is part of our sustainable future.

So this chapter briefly considers how these elements might be assembled to form a coherent system, one which might enjoy the confidence of the community and inspire individuals and communities to describe and design their own careers and future plans in a more positive light. One where albatross chicks feed on oily fish rather than regurgitated plastic; one where the elderly feel valued and respected rather than lonely and isolated; one where the vulnerable are nurtured, protected and supported to live fulfilling lives, are viewed as assets and inverse care law winners because of what they can offer and teach us, and we may become frail and vulnerable ourselves as our lives unfold. At its centre this system needs to redefine the inverse care law [1] to become a care law where the resources applied are directly correlated with needs and used to maximise the potential locked up in every member of the community.

RESPONSIBLE CITIZENSHIP

Although responsible citizenship is a concept most fully described and studied in the education world as "active citizenship" and internationally as a community development theme, it does have great resonance in the culture, history and development of welfare services in the UK.

From the time of the crusades – with the Red Cross's association with the order of the Knights Templar through to the District Nursing Association – the voluntary sector has been a key component of British welfare provision before the birth of the NHS and welfare state. It would be fair to assert that without this heritage of sustaining communities, the emergence of the NHS Mk 1 and the modern welfare state would have been impossible. The elements are integral and remain deeply ingrained in our social culture.

The Wanless report [2] discussed a "fully engaged" scenario where individuals take more responsibility for their own health. In NHS Mk 2, *responsible citizenship builds on this fully engaged scenario to build the new welfare system around the commitment of citizens to take responsibility for their own health and to actively support the system through which communities take responsibility for the welfare of local people. This is the new welfare paradigm underpinning the new social compact this vision is describing.*

- Examples of how this becomes central to the working of the new system include individuals holding and controlling their own lifelong health record, with it evolving from the current medical, dental, out-of-hours, nursing and social care record systems. This biographical record will inform all the individual's consultations with welfare providers and also contain letters, pathology and radiology results and agreed treatment escalation plans (TEPs), power of attorney details, living wills and a statement reflecting the social compact (i.e. the rights and responsibilities through which our lives and these plans and stories flourish). This needs therefore to become the individual's "log book" rather than just their clinical record. This builds on work from Australia [4] where individual people control access to their summary care records including parts of their GP, hospital, pharmacy, radiology and pathology details, and this model has been adopted in several other places including Austria and Nordic countries. The consequence will be that every consultation between the citizen and the new service will be informed by and contribute to their log book, minimising the major risk of the current dissonant system where multiple records tied to organisational boundaries inhibit rather than direct care provision.
- People being supported to *volunteer* to provide care, skills and time for the benefit of local people. CQC has seen excellent schemes in some communities where, with support and coordination, high-quality welfare provision can become a reality in partnership with volunteers. However, too often this has been in communities whose needs are not extreme. With the increased leisure available in the digital world and the current epidemics of loneliness, and frail elderly isolation, this model of empowered responsible citizenship has much to offer. Examples of really engaging and supportive schemes [3] have been found on CQC inspections, but are too frequently locally developed, to meet a particular identified need, rather than planned to address the vagaries of the inverse care law towards building a healthier community.
- The approach to social cohesion this envisages has other positive potential benefits – from supporting intergenerational and sectarian understanding, to offering a more positive future to young people growing up in the community and to the vulnerable (such as people with disabilities) who can become valued as members of the community with experience to offer as well as needs to be met. This is not the place to extend this vision into the world of social capital (sustainable housing schemes, community learning projects, etc.), but this has to be seen as the direction of travel in this liberated, "digital" world – not just a digital IT world but rather a digitally enabled, community approach.
- In NHS Mk 1, decision-making power, both about clinical practice and about organisational direction and management, has been held in professional hands (i.e. doctors run doctors surgeries, opticians run opticians shops) or by "corporate" provides (Vision Express and Virgin healthcare for example), or through local authorities (social services or NHS community trusts providing community nursing, for example). These governing arrangements no longer meet the needs of the community as we move into the digital world. In NHS Mk

2, responsible citizenship will require us to move beyond passive participation as "patients" to include the opening up of the governing arrangements so as to hold the clinical professionals and executive corporate management to account for the safety, quality and effectiveness of their performance. This sees the important role of the Care Quality Commission in holding provider organisations to account reinforced and embedded. In the field of education, parent governors have fulfilled this function for many years, and in almost every other sector of business or national life, non-executive directors have an important role in holding the executive to account [5]. This will mean that the organisation providing home-based care will need to move beyond current arrangements such as *patient participation groups* and *Leagues of Friends* to share power in the organisation in ways that make the system more trustworthy more accountable and more open to public scrutiny. The resilience of such "social enterprise" is also more assured given the breadth of social capital involved and its sustainability. In a rapidly changing world the power involved will be greater given the broader reach of this "welfare" paradigm. A further aspect of this needs to be considered. Quality improvement in NHS Mk 1 has been the responsibility in recent times of NHS Improvement, but it has no remit to support quality improvement in general practice or the primary care sector. This is a gap which should not be allowed to continue. Rather CQC findings should inform and support an expanded role for the NHS Modernisation Agency in NHS Mk 2. There will be a need for NHS Improvement to enhance its capacity and capability for this additional responsibility. NHS Mk 1 has lost much of its corporate memory of primary care in recent years. It will not be easy to replace it, but it is essential – to support the development of NHS Mk 2.

REDEFINED PROFESSIONALISM FROM PATERNALISM TO PARTNERSHIP

We have already discussed how the role of members of professional groups is changing as a result of how their relationship with the users of the services they provide has evolved [6]. In the digital world of NHS Mk 2, universal access to data and information liberates us all from relying on a professional "body of knowledge". Now most patients who consult me can be expected to have googled their symptoms and decided what they want me to do. In the same way I no longer need a huge library of learned texts to found my professional practice on; the library of knowledge is now accessible on my PC, in my consulting room and via my mobile phone whenever and wherever I am consulting.

In this new world the trust and respect membership of the medical and caring professions retain relies on the following:

- How power is held in the relationship between carer and citizen. If access to treatment (or gatekeeping) is controlled by the professional and this is valued by the customer, then it is empowering. However, if the customer seeks to buy favour by bribing the gatekeeper with presents or subsidised education (as the pharmaceutical industry has done for much of the NHS Mk 1 era), then it becomes demeaning. A therapeutic relationship requires both parties to trust each other, respect what each brings to the issue and acknowledge their interdependency. Professional partnerships, such as those between GPs in a practice, has always been reliant on trust between the partners, agreement on their responsibilities and mutual support. Now that partnership needs to expand to encompass the relationship between responsible citizens and clinical professionals.

- The roles which doctors, nurses, pharmacists and other professional groups play in the provision of care in NHS Mk 2 is likely to be very different from the roles they trained for and have provided in NHS Mk 1. All professional groups are affected by this, but I shall focus particularly on general practitioners, with the effects on nursing, pharmacists, dentists, opticians and other groups being similarly in transition. In NHS Mk 1 general practitioners have not only been independent medical advisers to everyone in the population, but also the employers of staff, provider of premises, directors of the provider organisation, gatekeeper to other sectors of care and holder of the lifelong medical record. Recently it has become increasingly difficult to recruit GPs and especially GP partners. Surveys and other qualitative research (**Exeter SW GP Survey 2017** [7]) have described the extent of this problem and explored the reasons why GPs perceive there are recruitment and retention problems:

1. GPs are feeling overworked and undervalued. The complexity of people's problems has risen with the increase in the numbers of the frail elderly, and reduction in the hospital length of stay. This is a concentration of power and responsibility for GPs and is bad news for them and for the people they look after.

2. At the same time the proportion of NHS resources available for home-based care has been in decline, as money has been diverted to shore up NHS becomes acute hospital trusts balance sheets. Inevitably this has put pressure on general practice profitability and therefore GP partners' take-home pay (this also applies to general dental practitioners, community pharmacists and opticians whose businesses have also been under pressure). These are the only unprotected pieces in the jigsaw; salaried doctors and other staff are all "protected" by their contracts of employment, community trust staff are all on salary bands, and dental and optician staff are mostly on employment contracts if they are owned by corporate providers. But the GPs, dentists and pharmacists I have spoken to tell me they have had to take several pay cuts over the last decade, averaging about a twenty percent reduction in take-home pay over that decade. This makes it difficult to persuade the next generation of potential partners to become a "profit-sharing partner" rather than remain on a salary. The NHS commitment to increasing investment in primary care is welcome, but the message is clear: investment without reform does not work. This risks being a "fix that fails" (see Chapter 7).

3. New GPs will have trained in posts where the shift pattern has offered them protection from the excessive workload experienced in the early years of NHS Mk 1. In the 1970s, it was common for junior doctors to be rostered to work over a hundred hours a week including working all weekend and alternate nights on top of a "normal" nine-to-five working week. GPs in training in recent years have been protected from excessive workload,

and even as salaried GPs their sessional commitment often limits their exposure to the level of demand experienced by GP partners who are left feeling exposed. In addition to this exposure to patient demand, GP partners often complain that they have ultimate responsibility when things go wrong as employers as well as directors of the business where clinical and corporate governance overlap.

The employment of additional nursing staff, pharmacists and trained healthcare assistants has been one response to the changing world and the CQC's inspection programme has shown how much safe, high-quality care can result. Systematic care of people with

- minor illness, such as upper respiratory tract infections;
- minor injury, such as cuts bruises and sprains;
- those long term conditions covered by detailed specifications (the Quality and Outcomes Framework [QOF], for example), such as diabetes and COPD;
- and the problems of frailty, cancer screening and immunisation

have all led to examples of excellent nursing practice. Clinical pharmacists often provide systematic supervision of people on long-term medication, and trained healthcare assistants (HCAs) show how skilled diagnostics and ongoing monitoring can contribute to effective long-term care of people with diabetes COPD and hypertension for example.

However, there remains a place for medical expertise as part of the picture of home-based care, and I offer this distillate (see Chapter 1 in addition): I would also reflect that the expansion of the clinical team promised in *The NHS Long Term Plan* [12] has to help the sector address issues such as:

- A comprehensive digital offering for all NHS populations – medicines supply, consultation, advice and health promotion for example.
- Breaking down barriers – direct access to our own biographical notes (see Chapter 8) but also the links with other sectors, like specialist and social care, where digital links through Skype or Lync are available now but rarely used to support and integrate care.
- Near-patient testing (or self-monitoring) – rapid diagnostics, home monitoring of anticoagulation, self-screening for cancer (such as cervical) are all used more widely around the world and could be really helpful in NHS Mk 2.
- Group sessions – such as for helping people cope with long-term conditions like diabetes, and chronic issues like anxiety alcohol or nicotine addiction.
- Moving beyond supplicant patient engagement and "patient participation groups" to empower citizens in support of active citizenship (see Partnership with nurses and phamacists).

However, the role of the *expert generalist* as the diagnostician in the team remains central for the foreseeable future, while others may diagnose diabetes from laboratory results. Diagnosis as a result of pattern recognition from history and examination is predominantly a skill learned through medical training and experience.

Vignette 1

SC, aged fifty-five, had always been fit – only known to me because of minor issues over the years – but now he had come back from his holiday early because of tiredness and myalgia, weight loss and sweats all happening in the last fortnight. Examination and initial tests were normal apart from a tachycardia and soft mitral systolic murmur. The medical registrar needed convincing, but SC was seen that day and subacute bacterial endocarditis confirmed. I next saw him a month later following a stormy journey around several specialist units and cardiac valve surgery; he has remained well ever since.

The family doctor is a *decision maker*. The team may all play their part in describing the picture, but medical training and experience adds value when decisions about clinical care and treatment are needed.

Vignette 2

JD, aged eleven, had fallen out big time with her parents, and following social services intervention was facing a case conference to decide about her ongoing care. We knew there were positives. Despite everything, the family had been a stable unit throughout her life. She was bright, attending school and keen to learn. Her younger sister really mattered to her and she was keen on boxing at the youth club. Attending the case conference, as the only participant other than her parents who had known her for more than a year and having heard the practice team's views, helped the conference decide to support the family at home.

The general practitioner can be a care manager in complex situations to support the making of difficult decisions.

Vignette 3

MJ was thirty-five and on more than twenty repeat medications for her rheumatoid arthritis, type 1 diabetes, complex pain syndrome, surgically induced menopause and depression. She needed further shoulder surgery but was really frightened about admission and a further twist to the worthlessness cycle that had blighted her whole life. Working with her, alongside our nurses, pharmacist, the specialist team at the hospital and her CPN over a period of about two years helped her reach her objective of having enough control of her co-morbidities and medication to find the strength to cope with surgery.

The family doctor is the provider of continuity of care and the link to bridge across organisational boundaries.

Vignette 4

CR had cystic fibrosis and had specialist care from a unit seventy miles away. As her family doctor I saw her at least twice a week and supported her home-based treatment, alongside a wonderful physiotherapist and nursing team. When she died ten years later in hospital, the weight of her biographical care helped her family accept her passing and move on. The team could reflect on their contribution to a care package which had supported her to the best life she could have had, and thirty years later her memory remains vibrant. Continuity of care can support the vulnerable to face their demons, to focus on the positives and trust enough to let go and fly.

Episodic, specialist care will be essential for those times when events emphasise and punctuate our biographies. But none of us are so secure in our identity that we can deny the importance of the contribution continuity becomes of care can make to high-quality, safe care.

MUTUALITY

Just as building societies were establishes as mutual benefit societies where the members recognise the mutual benefit to savers and borrowers involved, so the underlying concept of NHS Mk 1 involved the mutual benefit to citizens of contributing through taxation while fit and able to, so as to benefit when in need. This concept of being mutually dependent on each other remains at the core of the vision for NHS Mk 2 and is at odds with the view that that we are all individually responsible for ourselves (see Chapter 9, e.g. regarding Margaret Thatcher's views on society) [13]. This mutuality extends to being part of a community – not just a community of common interest but a community held together by the glue of cohesion and interdependency, where volunteering and contributing to the mutual benefit of each other is vital to sustaining a national welfare service which provides for the health and welfare needs for all members of the community. This does not preclude the need for financial contributions based on ability to pay to top-up tax funding, but it goes beyond basing the service simply on financial resources to an acceptance that tax is not a bottomless pit. In modern times with all the benefits of the digital world – increased leisure, more control of our own lives and relief from the drudgery of servitude and heavy manual labour – we have to develop a new social contract or compact to underpin our NHS Mk 2, a contract where citizenship involves contributing to the community, not just by paying taxes but by the expectation that contributing our time and energy to the benefit of those in the community who require it, has real value. We will all need care when we are older, we will have sickness and need to be cared for, we will have health problems and need treatment. And we all have expertise, skills and time to contribute to this new social contract. I call it "mutuality" (see Chapter 8), just like the mutual benefit involved in traditional building societies and the mutual benefit underpinning the housing association movement and the health and welfare care systems in the world before NHS Mk 1. Somehow the post-war welfare state has moved away from this concept of mutuality, but the CQC inspection programme in general practice has highlighted outstanding practices illustrating what might be achieved by a return to mutuality.

Vignette 5

- The practice in Weston-super-Mare, which cared for a large number of really vulnerable people receiving residential detox care which, realising the need within the community for fresh fruit and vegetables established a stall in their reception area.
- Inclusion Health in Leicester where the needs of the most socially isolated – asylum seekers and refugees – are addressed through a mutual benefit organisation (a social enterprise).
- A group of practices in rural North Devon who developed strong links with their local community – health education in schools, volunteer befriending and transport schemes, social prescribing and carer-support programmes.
- A farming area in the peak district the where mental health consequences of isolation were tackled by community support rather than medication.
- A large new housing estate in Buckinghamshire is home to many young families. Their relative social isolation is tackled by community engagement – from infant feeding problems to postnatal depression, bedwetting to domestic violence – all without adequate health visiting but as an outreach service from the local GP practice.

Identification, support and care from community resources are common themes in the examples drawn from very different communities but all looking inward to their own resources to help address the problems they face.

ORGANISATIONAL INTEGRATION

While initiatives like "new models of care", "accountable care organisations and systems", "general practice at scale", "integrated care systems" and "primary care networks" are all seen as attractive developments to increase the efficiency of NHS management within a given locality. In this vision of NHS Mk 2 (the national welfare service) it is the efficiency of care provision which drives integration. In our current disintegrated "out-of-hospital" health and welfare sector, coordination and continuity of care is undervalued. There is no common care record to aid communication and care planning, there is no effective commissioning of care to ensure safety and promote quality, and the people who risk getting the worst care are those who need the best.

Vignette 6

AW, aged eighty-six, had been transferred from the acute to the community hospital after admission with pneumonia. The out-of-hours GP team was asked to review him on a Sunday evening because he was "deteriorating". He was taking oseltamvir because there were six cases of flu on the ward, his renal function was poor (glomerular filtration rate [GFR] about 20 mL; normal is over 60 mL), he was hypotensive (low blood pressure), with poor oxygen saturation and was slightly confused. He had three large folders of care records – from the acute hospital, community team and GP hospital care records – but there was no access to his biographical GP record system. Review of his medical needs was made more difficult by the disintegrated and uncoordinated way in which the needs of this sick and vulnerable man were being addressed and the lack of a unified biographical care record.

The CQC regards *flexibility choice and continuity of care* as key criteria for rating the responsive domain when it inspects primary care providers [8] and has noted many examples of "good" or "outstanding" practice in this area. But in none of the reports I have seen, has the care of people throughout their care journey been effectively coordinated, let alone reflected their informed choice, in any way flexed to meet their needs and through care arrangements promoting continuity of care by clinicians or teams with ongoing responsibility for care. Often, skilled, caring and experienced staff, including those I have interviewed for the preceding vignettes, are wonderful people frustrated by trying to provide good care despite the circumstances.

In this vision, organisational integration is driven by *function, form and fuel*, as described earlier. But the design will need to be built around, and driven by, the needs of responsible citizens (and their vulnerable, weaker family members) for access to high-quality safe care rather than by organisational design, such as the refreshed GP partnership model advocated by Watson's recent review [9]. This review, excellent though it is in many ways, fails to address the issues raised above by "responsible citizenship" and the need for a new relationship between citizens and the Mk 2 national welfare service with power shifting towards the community and away from the professional paradigms. This requires provider organisations to be redesigned accordingly to promote integration "by design".

The function of the organisation providing care in the home-based sector in this NHS Mk 2 digital world will be to support every individual to maximise their health and welfare, to maximise the control they have over their lives and to ensure that care within the organisation is guided by the "golden thread" of every individual citizen's "story". To achieve this functionality, the integrated care organisation will need to span tribal territories, encompassing the medical, nursing, pharmaceutical, dental, optical, social care and informal care paradigms in ways that support rather than prevent coordinated care and promote individual autonomy and maturity rather than patient dependency.

LONG-TERM PLAN FOR THE NHS

Commenting on the recently published *Long-Term Plan* for the NHS requires that same consideration of form function and fuel [8–10].

1. *Form*: Moves towards providing primary care at scale covering populations of 30,000–50,000 are welcome but seem to be stuck in the "old medical model" of general practice plus community nursing without considering the consequences

of the issues raised in earlier chapters, e.g. the *empowered patient, mutuality* and *redefined professionalism* but also the issues of governance, openness and accountability in any primary care provider organisation. In moves towards practice at scale there is also the risk that personal care will suffer due to a weakening of personal responsibility.

2. *Function*: The plan provides an excellent framework for the development of the sector as the primary provider; transferring outpatient care from hospital, strengthening maternity and mental health provision and a focus on genetic healthcare are all going to shift the functions of the sector. Associated plans to reform primary care contracts [11] initially focusing on the Quality and Outcomes Framework and immunisation are also welcome but fall short of the agenda spelt out earlier to replace the national contracts and introduce a more local framework which addresses the needs of the local community and the local health economy while respecting the national perspective. The needs of some groups has not been focussed on sufficiently in recent years, including those with long-term conditions not included in the QOF arrangements, such as those with multiple sclerosis, poor hearing or vision, arthritis sufferers and those with congenital abnormalities (birth defects). All communities will have people with all of these and other problems that need to be appreciated, valued and addressed. About half of all adults are taking medication for long-term health issues, and all of us have health issues as part of our genetic inheritance and our own life experiences. All of these issues deserve more attention.

3. *Fuel*: The commitment of resources behind the plan is long overdue and welcome. But as pointed out earlier, money is not the only fuel required. Staffing and workforce issues have been weak for a long time and the vision of the plan is weak about this. Rather the new approach to professionalism described earlier is required to inspire people to commit their careers to working in the sector, spanning social as well as healthcare.

So, while welcome, the *Long-Term Plan* is too adherent to the current predominant paradigms and designs to reflect the realities of modern life: the digital world, the liberated and empowered citizen, and the need for a new social compact to inspire ongoing commitment to the NHS Mark 2 described earlier.

REFERENCES

1. Hart JT. 1971. The inverse care law. *Lancet* 297:405–12. https://www.thelancet.com/journals/lancet/article/PIIS0140-6736(71)92410-X/fulltext. Osler report Wood. 2009. https://core.ac.uk/download/pdf/2748417.pdf.
2. Wanless D. 2002. Securing our future health: Taking a long-term view. HM Treasury, London.
3. Gilburt H, Buck D and South J. 2018. Volunteering in general practice: Opportunities and insights. King's Fund. https://www.kingsfund.org.uk/publications/volunteering-general-practice.

4. Zhou N. 2018. My Health Record privacy framework 'identical' to failed UK scheme, experts says. *Guardian*, July 18. https://www.theguardian.com/australia-news/2018/jul/22/my-health-record-identical-to-failed-uk-scheme-privacy-expert-says.
5. Committee on the Financial Aspects of Corporate Governance. 1992. *The financial aspects of corporate governance [Cadbury Report]*. Gee Professional Publishing, London.
6. Hart T. 1988. *A New Kind of Doctor: The General Practitioner's Part in the Health of the Community*. Merlin Press, London.
7. Fletcher E, Abel GA, Anderson R et al. 2017. Quitting patient care and career break intentions among general practitioners in South West England: Findings of a census survey of general practitioners. *BMJ Open* 7:015853.
8. GP provider handbook. 2015. https://www.cqc.org.uk/guidance-providers/gps.
9. Watson N (chair). GP partnership review: Final report. 2019. https://cached.offlinehbpl.hbpl.co.uk/NewsAttachments/PGH/gp-partnership-review-final-report1.pdf.
10. Siddique H. 2019. Long term plan for NHS England 'undeliverable' amidst staffing crisis. *Guardian*, January 7. https://www.theguardian.com/society/2019/jan/07/long-term-plan-for-nhs-england-undeliverable-amid-staffing-crisis.
11. Lind S. 2019. New GP contract to mandate practices to join primary care networks. *Pulse*, January 7. http://www.pulsetoday.co.uk/home/finance-and-practice life-news/new-gp-contract-to-mandate-practices-to-join-primary-care-networks/20038055.article.
12. NHS. 2019. *NHS Long Term Plan*. https://www.england.nhs.uk/long-term-plan/.
13. Is society dead? *Independent*, 2016. https://www.Independent.co.uk/euro/uk/politics/society-dead-in7474856.html.31.10.2016.

Glossary

accountability: In ethics and governance, accountability is answerability, blameworthiness, liability and the expectation of account giving [1]. As an aspect of governance, it has been central to discussions related to problems in the public sector, and non-profit and private (corporate) and individual contexts. In leadership roles, accountability is the acknowledgment and assumption of responsibility for actions, products, decisions and policies including the administration, governance and implementation within the scope of the role or employment position and encompassing the obligation to report, explain and be answerable for resulting consequences.

In governance, accountability has expanded beyond the basic definition of "being called to account for one's actions". It is frequently described as an account-giving relationship between individuals, e.g. "A is accountable to B when A is obliged to inform B about A's (past or future) actions and decisions, to justify them, and to suffer punishment in the case of eventual misconduct". Accountability cannot exist without proper accounting practices; in other words, an absence of accounting means an absence of accountability.

ACO (accountable care organisation): A model of healthcare provision where a provider, or group of providers, takes responsibility for the healthcare provision of an entire population. There is no fixed definition of an ACO, but the organisation usually receives an annual, capitated budget to deliver contractually agreed health outcomes.

ACS (accountable care system): A system of healthcare provision which is intended to be integrated, and in particular to merge the funding of primary care with that for hospital care, therefore providing incentives to keep people healthy and out of hospital. It has features in common with accountable care organisations.

adaptive learning: Adaptive learning, also known as *adaptive teaching*, is an educational method which uses computer algorithms to orchestrate the interaction with the learner and deliver customised resources and *learning* activities to address the unique needs of each learner.

advocate: A person who puts a case on someone else's behalf.

aetiology: The study of the causes of disease.

aligned: To bring oneself into agreement with someone or someone's ideas; to associate oneself with someone or someone's cause. (Example sentence: She sought to align herself with the older members.)

analogy: A comparison between one thing and another, typically for the purpose of explanation or clarification.

analysis: The process of breaking a complex topic or substance into smaller parts in order to gain a better understanding of it. The technique has been applied in the study of mathematics and logic since before Aristotle (384–322 BC), though analysis as a formal concept is a relatively recent development.

anatomy: In its broadest sense, anatomy is the study of the structure of an object, in this case the *human body*. *Human anatomy* deals with the way the parts of *humans*, from molecules to bones, and how they interact to form a functional unit. Thus, anatomy and physiology are separate but complementary studies of how an organism works.

ANP (advanced nurse practitioner): A level of nursing that usually requires a master's level course of study or qualification.

AO (accountable officer): Individual with responsibility, who is held to account for performance.

APMS (alternative provider medical services): A form of contract for primary care services awarded and managed by local commissioners. Designed to meet specific local needs unmet by existing local GMS or PMS contracts.

apothecary: Apothecary is one term for a medical professional who formulates and dispenses materia medica to physicians, surgeons and patients. The modern pharmacist has taken over this role. In some languages and regions, the word "apothecary" is still used to refer to a retail pharmacy or a pharmacist who owns one.

appraisal: The formal structured process for a person to reflect on his or her work and to consider how his or her effectiveness might be improved.

archetype: The concept of an archetype appears in areas relating to *behaviour, historical psychological theory* and *literary analysis*. An archetype can be:

1. A statement, pattern of behaviour, a *prototype*, a "first" form or a main model which other statements, patterns of behaviour, and objects copy, emulate or "merge" into. (Frequently used informal synonyms for this usage include "standard example", "basic example", and the longer form "archetypal example". Mathematical archetypes often appear as "canonical examples".)
2. A *Platonic philosophical idea* referring to pure *forms* which embody the fundamental characteristics of a thing in Platonism.
3. A collectively inherited unconscious idea, pattern of thought, image, etc. that is universally present, in individual psyches, as in *Jungian psychology*.
4. A constantly recurring symbol or motif in literature, painting or mythology. (This usage of the term draws from both *comparative anthropology* and from *Jungian archetypal theory*). In various seemingly unrelated cases in classic storytelling, media, etc., characters or ideas sharing similar traits recur.

Archetypes are also very close analogies to instincts in the sense that the impersonal and inherited traits that present and motivate human behaviour long before any consciousness develops [1]. They also continue to influence feelings and behaviour even after some degree of consciousness develops later.

arrogance: (1) Exaggerating or disposed to exaggerate one's own worth or importance often by an overbearing manner an arrogant official. (2) Showing an offensive attitude of superiority, proceeding from or characterised by arrogance or an arrogant reply.

assurance: A positive declaration intended to give confidence. (Example sentence: He received assurances of support for the project.) Promise or pledge; guaranty; surety. (Example sentence: He gave his assurance that the job would be done.) Full confidence; freedom from doubt; certainty; to act in the assurance of success.

audit: The systematic measurement of performance and implementation of change against one or more predefined criteria against a standard until that standard is achieved or until a new standard is set.

Augean stables: From Hercules' fifth labor: Cleaning the Augean stables in a single day. The expression to "clean the Augean stables" is sometimes used in literature to describe a very difficult and unpleasant job, and is an example of Hercules not being given a trial of strength as a labour but rather a task which required thought and planning – using his thinking skills to devise a solution which had not been considered before. This is an example from Greek Mythology of lateral thinking or "thinking outside the box".

austerity: A political–economic term referring to policies that aim to reduce government budget deficits through spending cuts, tax increases or a combination of both. Austerity measures are used by governments that find it difficult to pay their debts.

autonomy: (1) The quality or state of being self-governing, especially the right of self-government. (Example sentence: The territory was granted autonomy.) (2) Self-directing freedom and especially moral independence or personal autonomy.

biographical care: *Biographical works* are usually non-fiction, but fiction can also be used to portray a person's life. One in-depth form of biographical coverage is called legacy writing. *Works* in diverse media, from literature to film, form the genre known as *biography*.

biopsychosocial model: Relating to, or concerned with the biological, psychological and social aspects in contrast to the strictly biomedical aspects of disease.

business model: A business model is the way an organisation creates, delivers and captures value, in economic, social, cultural or other contexts. The process of business model construction and modification is also called *business model innovation* and forms a part of business strategy.

capacity: The role or function someone is performing. While we usually define capacity as in how much something can hold, it also means the ability or power to do, experience or understand something.

capitalism: An economic system in which private individuals or businesses own capital goods. The production of goods and services is based on supply and demand in the general market (known as a market economy) rather than through central planning (known as a planned economy or command economy).

caring: (adjective) If someone is caring, they are affectionate, helpful and sympathetic. (Example sentence: He is a lovely boy, very gentle and caring.) Synonyms: compassionate, loving, kindly, warm. "Caring" is one of the five key domains that the CQC rates on all its inspections. The key criteria it considers looks beyond the provision of kind and compassionate to consider issues such as empowerment. Are people empowered and supported, where necessary, to use and link with support networks and advocacy, so that it will have a positive impact on their health, care and well-being [1]?

catalyst: A substance that increases the rate of a chemical reaction without itself undergoing any permanent chemical change; a person or thing that precipitates an event.

cathartic: Providing psychological relief through the open expression of strong emotions; causing catharsis.

CCG (clinical commissioning group): The primary care–led organisations set up by the Health and Social Care Act 2012 to organise and commission the delivery of National Health Services in England.

CF (cystic fibrosis): An inherited condition causing severe lung disease and intestinal problems.

clinical governance: The framework through which National Health Service organisations and their staff are accountable for the quality of patient care, or through which staff and patients are assured that their care provider is trustworthy.

clinical pharmacy: The branch of pharmacy in which clinical pharmacists provide direct patient care that optimises the use of medication and promotes health, wellness and disease prevention.

coherent: If an argument, set of ideas or a plan is coherent, it is clear and carefully considered, and each part of it connects or follows in a natural or reasonable way.

cohesion: The sticking together of particles of the same substance.

commissioning: The planning and purchasing of health services.

communism: A philosophical, social, political and economic ideology and movement whose ultimate goal is the establishment of a communist society, which is a socioeconomic order structured upon the ideas of common ownership of the means of production and the absence of social classes, money and the state.

communitarianism: A philosophy that emphasises the connection between the individual and the community. Its overriding philosophy is based upon the belief that a person's social identity and personality are largely moulded by community relationships, with a smaller degree of development being placed on individualism.

community: A group of people who share something in common. You can define a community by the shared attributes of the people in it and/or by the strength of the connections among them. You need a bunch of people who are alike in some way, who feel some sense of belonging or interpersonal connection.

co-morbidity: Coexistence of a disease or diseases in an individual which independently and synergistically affect the individual's quality of life.

complex systems: Systems incorporating multiple components and multiple interactions that can lead to non-linear and unpredictable rather than simple linear cause-and-effect reactions to stimuli.

confidence: Full trust; belief in the powers, trustworthiness or reliability of a person or thing. (Example sentence: We have every confidence in their ability to succeed.) Belief in oneself and one's powers or abilities; self-confidence; self-reliance; assurance. (Example sentence: His lack of confidence defeated him.)

confounding variable: A variable, other than the independent variable, that you're interested in that may affect the dependent variable. This can lead to erroneous conclusions about the relationship between the independent and dependent variables.

consanguinity: The fact of being descended from the same ancestor; sharing genetic heritage, having genes in common.

contractor: A person who provides their skills or services for a limited period of time. An *independent contractor* is a person, business, or corporation that provides goods or services under a written contract or a verbal agreement. Unlike employees, independent contractors do not work regularly for an employer but work as required, when they may be subject to law of agency. As compared to employees, contractors have more control over their hours and rate of pay for their services.

CQC (Care Quality Commission): The independent regulator responsible for the quality and safety of all health and social care services in England.

criticism: The practice of judging the merits and faults of something. The judger is called a critic. To engage in criticism is to criticise. One specific item of criticism is called a criticism or critique. Criticism is an evaluative or corrective exercise that can occur in any area of human life.

culture: The way of life of groups of people, meaning the way they do things. An integrated pattern of human knowledge, belief and behaviour. The outlook, attitudes, values, morals, goals, and customs shared by a society. Excellence of taste in the fine arts and humanities is known as high culture.

deference: The condition of submitting to the espoused, legitimate influence of one's superior or superiors. Deference implies a yielding or submitting to the judgment of a recognised superior, out of respect or reverence.

demography: The study of human populations, usually statistical and describing the population's characteristics – age, sex, ethnic background, employment status, etc.

desertification: A type of land degradation in dry lands involving loss of biological productivity caused by natural processes or induced by human activities. It is caused by a variety of factors, such as through climate change and through the overexploitation of soil through human activity.

diagnosis: *Medical diagnosis* (abbreviated Dx or D$_s$) is the process of determining which disease or condition explains a person's symptoms and signs. Often, one or more *diagnostic* procedures, such as medical tests, are also done during the process.

dialogue: A conversational exchange between two people. Most part of a **dialogue** includes questions and answers, requests and information. *Dialogue* is for purpose. *Conversation* is talking between two or more persons.

dichotomy: A division or contrast between two things that are or are represented as being opposed or entirely different.

digital: Describes electronic technology that generates, stores and processes data in terms of two states: positive and non-positive. A modem is used to convert the digital information in your computer to analogue signals for your phone line and to convert analogue phone signals to digital information for your computer.

disability: In the context of a health experience a disability is any restriction or lack (resulting from an impairment) of ability to perform an activity in the manner or within the range considered normal for the population.

discussion: The activity in which people talk about something and tell each other their ideas or opinions.

dispensing: Authorised or qualified to develop and provide medicine.

effectiveness: A measure of the benefit resulting from an intervention for a given health problem under usual conditions or clinical care for a particular group. As one of the five key domains reviewed by the CQC during its inspection programme, the focus is on improving outcomes and usually relies heavily on quantitative assessments, such as the Quality and Outcomes Framework (see *QOF*).

efficiency: The ratio of the useful work performed by a machine or in a process to the total energy expended or heat taken in. Efficiency is the ability to avoid wasting materials, energy, efforts, money, and time in doing something or in producing a desired result. In a more general sense, it is the ability to do things well, successfully and without waste.

egalitarian: Believing in or based on the principle that all people are equal and deserve equal rights and opportunities.

emancipation: The fact or process of being set free from legal, social or political restrictions; liberation.

empowerment: The process of becoming stronger and more confident, especially in controlling one's life and claiming one's rights.

encephalitis: Inflammation of the brain, caused by infection or an allergic reaction.

endowment: A donation of money or property to a non-profit organisation, which uses the resulting investment income for a specific purpose. Most endowments are designed to keep the principal amount intact while using the investment income for charitable efforts.

enfranchisement: The giving of a right or privilege, especially the right to vote.

entropy: A thermodynamic quantity representing the unavailability of a system's thermal energy for conversion into mechanical work, often interpreted as the degree of disorder or randomness in the system.

epidemiology: The study of the distribution and determinants of health-related states or events in specified populations, and the application of this study to control of health problems.

epigenetics: In biology, epigenetics is the study of heritable phenotype changes that do not involve alterations in the DNA sequence. The Greek prefix *epi-* implies features that are "on top of" or "in addition to" the traditional genetic basis for inheritance.

episodic: Containing or consisting of a series of separate parts or events.

escalation plan: A set of procedures set in place to deal with potential problems in a variety of contexts. In a call centre, for example, an escalation plan specifies measures to be implemented when unexpected strain or an increased level of stress is placed upon the centre.

essence: The intrinsic nature or indispensable quality of something, especially something abstract, which determines its character.

evidence-based healthcare/medicine: Systematic use of evidence derived from published research.

evolutionary: Relating to or denoting the process by which different kinds of living organisms are believed to have developed from earlier forms.

expert generalism: The term *expert-generalist* was coined by Orbit Gadiesh. He defined an expert-generalist as someone who has the ability and curiosity to master and collect expertise in many different disciplines, industries, skills, topics, capabilities, etc. Expert generalism has picked up in popularity of late.

fanaticism: A belief or behaviour involving uncritical zeal or with an obsessive enthusiasm. Philosopher George Santayana defines fanaticism as "redoubling your effort when you have forgotten your aim". The fanatic displays very strict standards and little tolerance for contrary ideas or opinions.

fascism: A form of far-right, authoritarian ultranationalism characterised by dictatorial power, forcible suppression of opposition, and strong regimentation of society and of the economy which came to prominence in early twentieth-century Europe.

flexibility: The quality of bending easily without breaking.

fundamental: A central or primary rule or principle on which something is based.

gatekeeper: A person who controls access to something, for example via a city gate.

general management: Duties and responsibilities include formulating policies, managing daily operations and planning the use of materials and human resources. This means that a general manager usually oversees most or all of the firm's marketing and sales functions, as well as the day-to-day operations of the business.

generative learning: A theory that involves the active integration of new ideas with the learner's existing schemata. Generative learning is, therefore, the process of constructing meaning through generating relationships and associations between stimuli and existing knowledge, beliefs and experiences.

gestation: The time between conception and birth. Though we're focussing on human gestation, this term applies more broadly to all animals.

globalisation: The process by which the world is becoming increasingly interconnected as a result of massively increased trade and cultural exchange. Globalisation has increased the production of goods and services.

GMC: National body with responsibility for accrediting medical training, maintaining a professional register of all doctors practising in the UK as well as setting and monitoring professional standards of practice.

GMS (general medical services): The detailed agreement between the UK government and general practitioners about the services they will provide under the National Health Service and what remuneration they will attract. Of the three forms of contracts agreed annually (the others being PMS and AMS), this one is negotiated nationally by the General Practitioners Committee from the British Medical Association and the Department of Health.

governance: Relates to "the processes of interaction and decision-making among the actors involved in a collective problem that lead to the creation, reinforcement, or reproduction of social norms and institutions". ... *Governance* is the way rules, norms and actions are structured, sustained, regulated and held accountable.

GP (general practitioner): Also known as a family doctor; doctors who are fully trained in both hospital posts and in general practice. They join the GP register managed by the General Medical Council and the National Performers List held by NHS England. They are normally self-employed. They provide general medical services, employ staff to help them and provide practice premises. They may become partners in a GP practice and be responsible for the care of people registered with the practice or be employed by a practice as a salaried doctor.

health promotion: The process of enabling people to increase control over their *health* and its determinants, and thereby improve their *health*.

heritage: The background from which one comes, or any sort of inherited property or goods. An example of heritage is a German ancestry. Another example of heritage is money left to a child in their parent's will.

holistic: Characterised by the treatment of the whole person, taking into account mental and social factors rather than just the symptoms of a disease.

hypothetical: A possibility, circumstance, statement, proposal, situation, etc. A tentative insight into the natural world; a concept that is not yet verified but that if true would explain certain facts or phenomena. Types: Hypothesis, possibility, theory.

ICS (integrated care system): In 2016, NHS organisations and local councils came together to form sustainability and transformation partnerships (STPs) covering the whole of England, and set out their proposals to improve health and care for patients. In some areas, a partnership will evolve to form an integrated care system, a new type of even closer collaboration. In an integrated care system, NHS organisations, in partnership with local councils and others, take collective responsibility for managing resources, delivering NHS standards and improving the health of the population they serve.

independent healthcare provider: A provider of healthcare services that is neither owned nor managed by the National Health Service. Such organisations may provide health services paid for by private individuals, by health insurance companies, by local authorities and by NHS Scotland.

in extremis: In extreme circumstances.

institutional capture: What happens to individuals when they become part of large organisations and how their behaviour is affected.

integrated: With various parts or aspects linked or coordinated.

intrusive inquiry: An inquisitive person is one who is bent on finding out all that can be found out by inquiry, especially of little and personal matters, and hence is generally meddlesome and prying. Inquisitive may be used in a good sense, though in such connection inquiring is to be preferred, as "an inquiring mind".

iterative process: A process for calculating a desired result by means of a repeated cycle of operations. An iterative process should be convergent, i.e., it should come closer to the desired result as the number of iterations increases.

leverage: (1) The ability to influence situations or people so that you can control what happens. Leverage is the force that is applied to an object when something such as a lever is used. (2) Use borrowed capital for (an investment), expecting the profits made to be greater than the interest payable.

liaison: Communication or cooperation which facilitates a close working relationship between people or organisations.

liberalism: A political and moral philosophy based on liberty, consent of the governed and equality before the law.

libertarian: A collection of political philosophies and movements that uphold liberty as a core principle. Libertarians seek to maximise political freedom and autonomy, emphasising freedom of choice, voluntary association and individual judgment.

LMC (local medical committee): Local representative committees of NHS GPs that represent their interests in their localities to the NHS health authorities. LMCs interact and work with, and through, the General Practitioners Committee as well as other branches of practice committees and local specialist medical committees in various ways, including conferences. *LDCs, LOCs and LPCs* perform similar roles for dentists, opticians and pharmacists, respectively.

LPA (lasting power of attorney): Allows you to give someone you trust the legal power to make decisions on your behalf in case you later become unable to make decisions for yourself. An *LPA for Health and Welfare* covers decisions about health and personal welfare. Continuing (financial) powers can be used by the attorney immediately after the power of attorney document has been registered. If the power of attorney is only to be used in the event of your incapacity, it must clearly state that the powers are not to be used until this happens. You may wish to add a statement about who should make this decision about your incapacity.

mastery: Comprehensive knowledge or skill in a particular subject or activity.

maturity: The quality or state of being mature, especially full development.

mental model: An explanation of someone's thought process about how something works in the real world. It is a representation of the surrounding world, the relationships between its various parts, and a person's intuitive perception about his or her own acts and their consequences.

mentoring: Mentorship is a relationship in which a more experienced or more knowledgeable person helps to guide a less experienced or less knowledgeable person. The mentor may be older or younger than the person being mentored, but he or she must have a certain area of expertise.

mindset: The established set of attitudes held by someone.

monitor: The sector regulator for health services in England that has a role to protect and promote the interests of patients. Also has the responsibility for improving services of patients. Does not have any responsibility for these functions in the primary care sector of the NHS.

morbidity: The impact of a disease that is not death; measures of morbidity include incidence and prevalence rates.

mortality (rates): Death; the number of deaths in an area as a proportion of the number of people in that area.

motivation: Derived from the word *motive* which means needs, desires, wants or drives within the individuals. It is the process of stimulating people to actions to accomplish the goals. In the work goal context, the psychological factors stimulating the behaviour can be desire for money or success.

MPC (Medical Practices Committee): A national committee which was tasked with ensuring an even spread of GPs across the country by encouraging movement from over-doctored areas to under-doctored areas.

mutual: A private organisation that is owned by its customers, policyholders or employees. Mutuals take several forms, including friendly societies, building societies and housing associations. Mutual love, however, means you can feel secure that you both love and are loved equally, and you and your partner are approximately equal in your energy for staying together. There are four major areas of mutuality that must be present if a relationship if it is to succeed and grow: love, benefit, trust and support.

need: The need for healthcare is the capacity to benefit from the care provided.

neonatal mortality: The proportion of live births who die within the first 28 days.

ONS (Office for National Statistics): The executive office of the UK Statistics Authority, a non-ministerial department which reports directly to the UK Parliament.

organisational development: The process used to ensure effective growth and longevity, and improve the overall effectiveness of an organisation through managing the behaviours of people within that organisation.

paradigm: A distinct set of concepts or thought patterns, including theories, research methods, postulates and standards for what constitutes legitimate contributions to a field.

partnership: A legal form of business operation between two or more individuals who share management and profits. The federal government recognises several types of partnerships. In a *general partnership*, the partners manage the company and assume responsibility for the partnership's debts and other obligations.

paternalism: The policy or practice on the part of people in authority of restricting the freedom and responsibilities of those subordinate to or otherwise dependent on them in their supposed interest.

patient participation group: Groups of volunteer patients of a practice with members of practice staff who meet regularly to discuss services and how they might be improved.

PEST (or PESTLE) analysis: An analysis of the political, economical, social and technological (and legal and environmental) factors or forces determining change.

physiology: The scientific study of the functions and mechanisms which work within a living system.

PMS (personal medical services): *PMS contracts* provide similar core medical services to GMS contracts but can also include extra health services that are considered to be "over and above" the usual core services, for example special clinics for homeless people in areas of high need. This contract type is negotiated and monitored locally between provider and commissioner.

policy: An overall statement of the aims of an organisation within a particular context.

pool arrangement: A contractual arrangement by which corporate shareholders agree that their shares will be voted as a unit. Therefore, a voting trust is created between a group of stockholders and the trustee to whom they transfer their voting rights.

populism: A political approach that strives to appeal to ordinary people who feel that their concerns are disregarded by established elite groups.

prevalence: The proportion of persons with a particular disease within a given population at a given time. *Point prevalence* is the prevalence at one single point in time.

Period prevalence is the proportion of persons with a particular disease over a specified period of time.

primary healthcare: First contact care provided by a range of healthcare professionals – nurses, dentists, pharmacists, optometrists and complementary therapists as well as doctors.

pro bono: Denoting work undertaken without charge, especially legal work for a client on low income.

profession(alism): A *profession* is a job at which someone works and for which they have had training. It is what they do to get money or a living. People often study for years to do their job. Sometimes "profession" only means learned professions, but sometimes the word may also be used for other jobs. For some, being professional might mean dressing smartly at work or doing a good job. For others, being professional means having advanced degrees or other certifications, framed and hung on the office wall. *Professionalism* encompasses all of these definitions.

prognosis: The possible outcomes of a disease or condition and the likelihood that each one will occur.

QOF (Quality and Outcomes Framework): The national primary care payment for performance (P4P) scheme in the United Kingdom.

reductionist: Analysing and describing a complex phenomenon in terms of its simple or fundamental constituents.

resilient: Able to withstand or recover quickly from difficult conditions.

respect: Due regard for the feelings, wishes or rights of others.

responsibility: Duty or obligation to satisfactorily perform or complete a task (assigned by someone, or created by one's own promise or circumstances) that one must fulfil, and which has a consequent penalty for failure.

responsiveness: The quality of being responsive; reacting quickly. As a quality of people, it involves responding with emotion to people and events. One of the five key domains which the CQC inspects on every inspection. But the CQC considers more than just the quality of the emotional response, it also considers how the organisation responds to the needs of the population it serves and the timeliness of that response [1].

revalidation: The process by which licensed doctors are required to demonstrate once every five years that they are up to date and fit to practice.

rhetoric: The art of persuasion, which along with grammar and logic, is one of the three ancient arts of discourse. Rhetoric aims to study the capacities of writers or speakers needed to inform, persuade or motivate particular audiences in specific situations.

safe(ty): By safe, we mean people are protected from abuse and avoidable harm. Abuse can be physical, sexual, mental or psychological, financial, neglect, institutional or discriminatory. One of the five domains the CQC always reviews on inspection to see to what extent the organisation ensures the safety of users of the service – be they vulnerable children through appropriate safeguarding arrangements or the whole population through ensuring staff are qualified and trained, and medicines are handled safely, for example [1].

SALT: Usually a specialist team based in hospital to advise on diet and treatment.

SEA (significant event analysis): A method of audit that involves systematic and detailed review of "significant" incidents identified by one or more of the practice team, reflecting systematically on what occurred with the team and making recommendations for improvement.

Shipman, Harold: English GP Harold Shipman was convicted of murdering 15 of his patients in 2000, and is thought to have killed up to 250 of his patients; this led to the Shipman Inquiry by Dame Janet Smith into the deaths.

Skype: Skype is a telecommunications application that specialises in providing video chat and voice calls between computers, tablets, mobile devices, the Xbox One console and smartwatches via the Internet. Skype also provides instant messaging services. Users may transmit text, video, audio and images. Theoretically available to all clinicians through their desktop computers – linked to their NHS email accounts – but in practice little used.

social enterprise: A commercial organisation that has specific social objectives that serve its primary purpose. Social enterprises seek to maximise profits while maximising benefits to society and the environment. Their profits are principally used to fund social programs.

socialism: Socialism encompasses a range of economic and social systems characterised by social ownership of the means of production and workers' self-management of enterprise, as well as the political theories and movements associated with such systems.

strategy: A plan of action designed to achieve a series of objectives. Strategy is important because the resources available to achieve these goals are usually limited. Strategy generally involves setting goals, determining actions to achieve the goals, and mobilising resources to execute the actions. A strategy describes how the ends (goals) will be achieved by the means (resources). Strategy can be intended or can emerge as a pattern of activity as the organisation adapts to its environment or competes. It involves activities such as strategic planning and strategic thinking.

supplicant: Can be a fervently religious person who prays to God for help with a problem, and it can also be someone who begs earnestly for something he or she wants. A younger brother entreating his sister to be allowed in her tree house could be described as a supplicant.

sustainability and sustainable development: The quality of causing little or no damage to the environment and therefore able to continue for a long time.

symmetry: Symmetry in everyday language refers to a sense of harmonious and beautiful proportion and balance. In mathematics, symmetry has a more precise definition and is usually used to refer to an object that is invariant under some transformations, including translation, reflection, rotation or scaling.

synthesis: The combination of components or elements to form a connected whole.

system: A set of interdependent and interacting elements, whether people organisations or processes that, together with the context in which they operate, seek to achieve a common aim.

systematic: Done or acting according to a fixed plan or system; methodical.

transactional (analysis): Transactional analysis is a psychoanalytic theory and method of therapy wherein social transactions are analysed to determine the ego state of the patient as a basis for understanding behaviour. In transactional analysis, the patient is taught to alter the ego state as a way to solve emotional problems.

transformation: The operation of changing (as by rotation or mapping) one configuration or expression into another in accordance with a mathematical rule, especially a change of variables or coordinates in which a function of new variables or coordinates is substituted for each original variable or coordinate.

trustworthy: Trustworthy is an adjective meaning able to be relied on. As an adjective, *reliable* means consistently good in quality or performance, able to be trusted. As a noun, reliable means someone or something with trustworthy qualities. Of course, trustworthy and reliable are synonyms when they refer to the same quality or performance.

vestigial: Being a small remaining part or amount. In medicine, used to describe something, especially a part of the body, that has not developed completely, or has stopped being used and has almost disappeared, for example a vestigial organ/limb/tail.

vignette: Definition, delineation, depiction, description, picture, portrait, portraiture, portrayal, rendering, sketch. Words related to vignette: account, anecdote, chronicle, narrative, report, story, tale, yarn. Demonstration, exemplification, illustration.

vituperative: Vituperative remarks are full of hate, anger or insults.

vocation: A type of work that you feel you are suited to doing and to which you should give all your time and energy, or the feeling that a type of work suits you in this way.

welfare: Statutory procedure or social effort designed to promote the basic physical and material well-being of people in need.

well-led: One of the five domains which the CQC reviews on inspection. By well-led, we mean that the leadership, management and governance of the organisation ensures the delivery of high-quality and person-centred care, supports learning and innovation, and promotes an open and fair culture. The key lines of enquiry considered cover issues such as capacity and capability of leaders; organisational culture; assigning and holding of responsibility; governance and openness.

REFERENCE

1. Care Quality Commission. 2019, April. How CQC monitors, inspects and regulates NHS GP practices. www.cqc.org.uk/GP. April 2019 provider handbook and key lines of enquiry.

Abbreviations

A&E	accident and emergency department
ACO	accountable care organisation
ACS	accountable care system
ANP	advanced nurse practitioner
AO	accountable officer
APMS	alternative provider medical services
BBC	British Broadcasting Corporation
BMA	British Medical Association
BMJ	*British Medical Journal*
BMS	Bachelor of Medical Science
CAMHS	Child and Adolescent Mental Health Services
CCG	clinical commissioning group
CF	cystic fibrosis
CHD	coronary heart disease
CPN	community psychiatric nurse
CQC	Care Quality Commission
DNCPR	do not attempt cardiopulmonary resuscitation
EC	executive council
ED	emergency department
FHSA	Family Health Services Authority
FPC	family practitioner committee
GMC	General Medical Council
GMS	general medical services
GP	general practitioner
ICA	integrated care assessment
ICS	integrated care system
IHR	individual healthcare record
IT	information technology
LMC	local medical committee
LPA	lasting power of attorney
MAU	medical assessment unit
MBA	Masters in Business Administration
Mk	Mark
MPC	Medical Practices Committee

NHS	National Health Service
NHSE	National Health Service Executive
NMC	new models of care
NMC	Nursing and Midwifery Council
ONS	Office for National Statistics
OT	occupational therapist
PCT	primary care trust
PEST (or PESTLE) analysis	political, economical, social and technological (and legal and environmental) analysis
PMS	personal medical services
QOF	Quality and Outcomes Framework
RCGP	Royal College of General Practitioners
RIP	rest in peace
SALT	speech and language therapy
SCIE	Social Care Institute for Excellence
SEA	significant event analysis
TB	tuberculosis
TSB	Trustee Savings Bank
UHW	University Hospital of Wales
UK	United Kingdom
USA	United States of America

Index

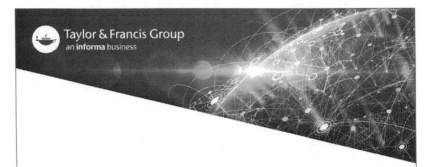